YOGA
BODY & MIND
HANDBOOK

WINNIPEG
MAY 1 1 2017
LIBRARY

D1536211

WITHDRAWN

Easy Poses
and Guided
Meditations

Perfect Peace
Wherever
You Are

YOGA
BODY & MIND
HANDBOOK

Jasmine
Tarkeshi

**SONOMA
PRESS**

Copyright © 2017 by Jasmine Tarkeshi

No part of this publication may be reproduced, stored in a retrieval
system, or transmitted in any form or by any means, electronic, mechanical,
photocopying, recording, scanning, or otherwise, except as permitted
under Section 107 or 108 of the 1976 United States Copyright Act, without the prior written permission of the publisher. Requests to the publisher
for permission should be addressed to the Permissions Department,
Sonoma Press, 918 Parker St., Suite A-12, Berkeley, CA 94710.

Limit of Liability/Disclaimer of Warranty: The publisher and the author make
no representations or warranties with respect to the accuracy or complete-
ness of the contents of this work and specifically disclaim all warranties,
including without limitation warranties of fitness for a particular purpose.
No warranty may be created or extended by sales or promotional materials.
The advice and strategies contained herein may not be suitable for every
situation. This work is sold with the understanding that the publisher is
not engaged in rendering medical, legal, or other professional advice or
services. If professional assistance is required, the services of a competent
professional person should be sought. Neither the publisher nor the author
shall be liable for damages arising herefrom. The fact that an individual,
organization, or website is referred to in this work as a citation and/or
potential source of further information does not mean that the author
or the publisher endorses the information the individual, organization,
or website may provide or recommendations they/it may make. Further,
readers should be aware that Internet websites listed in this work may have
changed or disappeared between when this work was written and when it
is read.

For general information on our other products and services or to obtain
technical support, please contact our Customer Care Department within
the United States at (866) 744-2665, or outside the United States at
(510) 253-0500.

Sonoma Press publishes its books in a variety of electronic and print for-
mats. Some content that appears in print may not be available in electronic
books, and vice versa.

TRADEMARKS: Sonoma Press and the Sonoma Press logo are trademarks
or registered trademarks of Arcas Publishing, a Callisto Media Inc. company
and/or its affiliates, in the United States and other countries, and may not be
used without written permission. All other trademarks are the property of
their respective owners. Sonoma Press is not associated with any product
or vendor mentioned in this book.

Illustrations © 2017 Ryan Johnson

Cover photo © Lumina/RG&B Images/Stocksy
Author photograph © Becca Henry

ISBN: Print 978-1-943451-56-2 | eBook 978-1-943451-57-9

This book is dedicated to my beautiful family,
whose support made writing this book possible,
as well as to my universal family, who I learn
from and practice with daily.

CONTENTS

INTRODUCTION

Welcome to *your* yoga practice. Whether you're new to yoga or rediscovering the practice, this guide will get you on the mat, moving, breathing, and meditating your way to a healthier, happier you.

Yoga is the simplest form of self-healing. I know this from my own experience and what I observe in my students. Almost anyone can enjoy yoga's benefits. You don't have to be in perfect shape or change your life to start your practice. You can do it anytime and anywhere. The point of yoga is not perfection. In fact, the first ancient *Yoga Sutra* says, "*Atha yoga anushasanam*," which means, "Now, the practice of yoga begins." The point is simply to begin.

In my yoga journey, I've found myself beginning again and again. As a dancer, in my teens, I practiced yoga solely for the physical benefits of increased strength and flexibility.

Then in my twenties, when struggling with self-destructive habits and the death of a partner, I took up yoga again by tapping into the mental, emotional, and spiritual benefits it offered. By studying the yogic texts and philosophy, I explored the deeper practices of meditation, *pranayama* (breathing techniques), and *mantra* (the repetition of sacred Sankrit sounds). These practices guided me to look within, rather than externally, for the peace and happiness I was searching for.

In my thirties, following hip and knee surgery, I returned for physical healing. My focus shifted toward conscious alignment and the stacking of bones and joints to achieve stability. I learned the blessings and work involved in even the simplest movements like standing, balancing, and sitting. Instead of trying to achieve complicated poses, this stage of my practice was all about having a curious beginner's mind and becoming a better teacher by listening.

I began yet again in my forties during pregnancy. Facing bed rest and a C-section, I was grateful for visualization, breathing, and meditative practices that kept me calm and centered. Postpartum healing, emotionally and physically, was slow and challenging, but my practice of acceptance and surrender was constant. As I got stronger and my practice grew more physical again, I snapped right back into pre-pregnancy shape—without even consciously trying.

A yoga practice isn't static, but rather something that grows with you as your body and mind change. As a busy mom, yoga studio owner, teacher, and writer, I need my practice today more than ever. I might practice for 15 minutes before my toddler wakes up or after she goes to sleep. I can also practice when I'm standing in the kitchen or sitting on an airplane. Yoga goes way beyond exercises on the mat. You can practice mindfulness all day long, and bring yoga into everything you do. Practicing yoga can relieve your physical, mental, and emotional tension. It can help you feel your best and live up to your highest potential.

My intention in writing this book is to guide you toward all the blessings of yoga: a tension-free body, a peaceful mind, a joyful spirit, an open heart, and a more authentic and fulfilling life. I start out by walking you through yoga's basic philosophy and practices. Then I show you how to adapt this ancient method of self-healing to your life. The book features different poses and routines that incorporate physical, breathing, and meditation exercises. You can mix up these routines to suit your needs and to keep your practice fresh and fun. I also explore ways for you to bring your practice off the mat through more mindful living. Finally, I explain the yogic concept of service and how to take the benefits out into the world.

Yoga has changed my life in so many ways. As a teacher, I've had the honor of witnessing my students' lives similarly transform through yoga. I'm excited to offer you the same chance. This book is all you need to start your journey to improved health, happiness, and peace of mind.

Now, your practice of yoga begins.

1

ONE

Mind and Body as One

What do you think of when you hear the word yoga? Perhaps you see an image of a beautiful, serene woman balancing on one leg at sunset. Or you see rows of young, perfectly synchronized athletic bodies in a well-lit yoga studio. But yoga is so much more than a trend or workout. It's a way of life that leads to inner peace and harmony. In fact, poses are just one small aspect of yoga. And anyone, regardless of body type or athletic ability, can reap the benefits of a yoga practice. Let's start with the basics.

What is Yoga?

Yoga originated thousands of years ago in India. In the Eastern world, yoga is treated as a spiritual practice for life. It's about more than the body; it includes the mind and spirit and how we conduct ourselves in the world.

The literal translation of the word *yoga* is "to yoke, join." It also means "discipline." Through the various translations, yoga is primarily understood to mean "union." In its ancient meaning, this union is between the individual soul with the universal soul, which leads to connection with all beings, nature, and the universe as a whole. Modern yogis translate this meaning into its simplest form: the union of the body and the mind. In this approach, the mind and the body aren't separate entities. They are one.

You don't have to practice yoga poses to understand this concept. Think about the relationship of your body and mind in your everyday life. If you're sad, your body will respond. You may curl up in your bed, slouch at your desk, or even cry. Conversely, you can change your physical state to alter your state of mind. If you're feeling low, going for a walk or dancing in your living room can make you feel better. This is yoga! It's more than just a set of poses you do to get a toned body. It's a way to join the mind and the body to improve every facet of life.

Yoga teaches us to be aware of our bodies and minds. In doing this, we learn to be fully present. This is done through the poses, breathing, and meditation. When you focus on movement, balance, and breathing, it can help you with other challenges in life.

Part of yoga is holding a pose even when it becomes uncomfortable. The pose may feel awkward or shaky, or cause your muscles to burn. By focusing on your breathing, you can get through the uncomfortable sensation. During an hour-long practice, little inconveniences like muscle fatigue or tightness will happen frequently. Each inconvenience is a lesson in how to react to the tougher times in life. When you can get through the uncomfortable poses that affect your body on the mat, your attitude toward the challenges in your life when off the mat will begin to shift as well.

Yoga teaches us how to tune in to our bodies so that we can make the best choices for our well-being, and therefore for the well-being of all. Yoga is a discipline for conscious living. This means that anything we do consciously is actually yoga.

A Brief History of Yoga

In the Western world, yoga may seem like a relatively new trend, but its roots stretch way back in ancient history. The first yogic scriptures were written in India between 1000 and 500 BC. They were hymns written in Sanskrit called the *Vedas*, which means "knowledge," and they focused mainly on the joining—or union—of the material and spiritual worlds through rituals and ceremonies. The Vedic sages, "seers" or "saints" who wrote the Vedas, connected the two worlds by concentrating for long periods of time, seeking to discover the root of their existence through the focus of the mind.

Later, sometime between the seventeenth and fifth centuries BC, the *Upanishads*, a huge collection of Hindu stories, presenting yoga's philosophy and practices, was published. This text continued the philosophy of the Vedas and acted as spiritual guides for applying the transcendental self to daily life. During this period, the *Bhagavad Gita* was also written; many yogis still use this parable to learn how to let go of the ego.

Next came what is known as the classical period of yoga. This period centers on Patanjali's *Yoga Sutras* and the idea that the mind and the body must be worked on separately through poses and meditation.

A few centuries after the *Yoga Sutras*, regarded as the "bible" of yoga, the post-classical period of yoga began, bringing more focus to the strengths and abilities of the body. Yoga masters of this time created a system of postures to challenge the body and prolong its life. This system evolved into Hatha yoga, and was the beginning of what we now recognize as the physical practice of yoga poses, or *asana*. This is where we first see asana and breathing practices described in detail along with their benefits in texts such as the *Hatha Yoga Pradipika* and the *Shiva Samhita*.

THE REWARDS OF YOGA

The rewards of yoga are plenty, and they tend to change over time. At first, yoga's benefits may seem strictly on the surface, like being able to touch your toes. Yet with time these benefits go much deeper. The more you practice yoga, the more you'll notice the rewards in your life, including:

- **A strong body, inside and out.** The physical practice of yoga not only strengthens and stretches your muscles. It can also lead to a stronger heart, increased lung capacity, and a more fluid lymphatic system.
- **A calm mind and reduced stress.** Yoga and modalities such as breathing exercises and meditation help drown out the outside world and allow you to focus on the moment, letting other worries drift away.
- **A sense of community.** Any time you participate in a shared experience, you develop a common purpose with others, which provides a sense of belonging.
- **Heightened concentration and clarity.** The focus required to move through the poses becomes second nature over time and will lead to greater focus off the mat.
- **Personal discovery.** Using the poses, or asanas, as a tool to access the mind, yoga takes you on an emotional, physical, and spiritual path of self-discovery.
- **Changing the world.** Gandhi's famous remark, "Be the change you wish to see in the world," is at the heart of yoga. A yogi feels at one with others and lives in a way that benefits others. A more peaceful, mindful you will radiate out to the people around you and the wider world.

In 1893, Swami Vivekananda, a great charismatic teacher and student of one of India's most beloved and enlightened teachers, Ramakrishna, landed on Western soil. He introduced yoga to the American public for the first time at the Parliament of Religions held in Chicago. He taught mostly about the mind, meditation, visualization, and Patanjali's Eight Limbs of Yoga (see below). But what endeared him to the West was his message of universal truth, which was so needed at the time. And so the modern period of yoga began. Since then, the method has taken root in the West, with millions of people practicing some type of yoga or meditation.

Today's yogis draw from all previous periods of yoga. Teachers still frequently reference ancient texts such as the *Bhagavad Gita* and the

EIGHT LIMBS OF YOGA

No matter how the physical practices of yoga evolve or change, the core philosophy does not. Patanjali, who is considered the father of the yogic philosophy, broke the practice down into what he called the Eight Limbs of Yoga:

1 *Yama*—Self-restraint. This pillar outlines five specific ways to practice self-restraint:
   * Do no harm (*ahimsa*)
   * Practice honesty (*satya*)
   * Do not steal (*asteya*)
   * Do not waste energy (*brahmacharya*)
   * Practice non-greed (*aparigraha*)
2 *Niyama*—How to act in the world. There are five ways to practice how to act:
   * Cleanliness (*saucha*)
   * Contentment (*santosha*)
   * Heat, or effort, to work through challenges (*tapas*)
   * Self-study (*svadhyaya*)
   * Acknowledgment that there is something bigger out there than ourselves (*Isvara Pranidhana*)
3 *Asana*—The physical postures of a yoga practice, or the poses.
4 *Pranayama*—The regulation of life force through the breath.
5 *Pratyahara*—The practice of withdrawing the mind from the senses.
6 *Dharana*—The ability to concentrate on one thing and let all else fall away.
7 *Dhyana*—Meditation.
8 *Samadhi*—The divine union of the individual with the universal, or moments of balance between mind and body.

Yoga Sutras. Modern yogis emphasize poses and ways to unite the body and mind with the breath. In fact, the dynamic yoga we know and practice today was innovated by the teacher known as the father of modern yoga, Krishnamacharya (1888–1988), as a blend of ancient poses and Western gymnastics and wrestling.

Asana

Asanas are the poses of yoga. These include well-known positions such as Downward-Facing Dog, Child's Pose, Plank Pose, and Upward-Facing Dog.

The original purpose of asana was to prepare the body to sit for long periods of time in meditation. The poses were used to relax the body and quiet the mind by focusing on one position instead of fidgeting and worrying. While you may not be ready to sit in meditation for hours on end (though you're certainly welcome to try!), the poses themselves are a form of meditation. When you move through the poses and focus on your body, you leave no room for your mind to wander. You may even hear asana referred to as "moving meditation."

Even the simplest asanas work in complex ways. Yoga poses require you to work against gravity and support the weight of your body in each position. Asanas also work in opposites: While you strengthen one part of your body, you stretch another. The phrase "*Sthira sukham asanam*" comes from one of

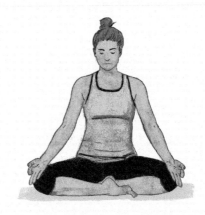

To begin, sit on the ground and cross your legs in front of you so your shins or ankles overlap. If this is uncomfortable, place a folded blanket or firm cushion under your sit bones. Sit up tall and close your eyes.

Next, do a body scan starting from your toes. Notice what you feel at each point in your body. Are your toes clenched? What about your knees—are they high in the air or close to the ground? Are they tense or resting comfortably? How about your hips? What do you feel there? Now continue moving up your body to your torso and your spine, then your shoulders, neck, head, and face. Observe where you feel at ease and where you're uncomfortable. Take note of these things and make little adjustments as needed.

If you take a moment out of your day to sit in Sukhasana and observe your body, you'll come in tune with its needs and discover a new way to focus your mind.

15

MIND AND BODY AS ONE

Patanjali's *Yoga Sutras* and is the definition of "asana." It basically means there's both strength and relaxation in the poses.

The asanas are also therapeutic and healing as they invigorate your internal organs, the digestive and endocrine systems, and the nervous system. In fact, many Western doctors now prescribe yoga for various ailments including back pain, sciatica, high blood pressure, anxiety, stress, depression, and more.

You don't have to do complex poses to experience the benefits of yoga. A simple asana, like Easy Pose (Sukhasana) (page 15), will do. (As you read through the book, you will notice that for some poses, I have provided Sanskrit translations for a pose or exercise name. Some others that have been developed in more recent times do not have Sanskrit names.)

OBSERVE YOURSELF

Yoga is most useful when you can translate the attention you bring to the poses to all parts of your life. One of the greatest lessons from the mat is to become aware of how you react to things. In the middle of a pose, those reactions come from physical sensations. You may discover a pose that feels really good for your body. This is a way to learn what your body needs and where to focus in your practice. Or you may find yourself in a pose that feels extremely challenging. Take note of your reactions. Settle into them as you hold the poses. This type of attention will help in your everyday life as triumphs or disappointments arise. Notice your reactions throughout the day. Can you sit with something uncomfortable, as you do on the mat, before you react? What does this feel like? What happens next?

Over time this will become second nature. By observing yourself, you'll be able to make mindful choices for your well-being regardless of the situation.

Breathing

The breath is what unites our mind to our body and life force. During practice, the breath helps warm up, nourish, and cleanse the body. It also quiets the mind by giving it something to focus on. When you work through the poses, you link the breath to your movements. For every move, you either inhale or exhale. This connection between the breath and the movement of the body is called *vinyasa*.

The breathing practices of yoga are called *pranayama*. *Prana* means "life force" and *ayama* means, "to extend or control." Ancient yogis believed we are born with a certain number of breaths, so slowing down the breath extends life.

The most common type of breathing in yoga is the Warrior's Breath, or *Ujjayi pranayama*. *Ujjayi* means "victorious," and in this context it relates to becoming victorious over your mind. The breath is controlled and steady. Breathe deeply in and out of your nose and focus on matching the length of your inhales to the length of your exhales.

Begin in Easy Pose (page 15), then take a moment to observe your natural breath. Don't try to change anything, just note what happens in your body. How does your chest rise and fall? Are your breaths quick? Deep or shallow?

Now gently close your mouth and slowly take a deep breath through your nose. As you breathe in, focus on allowing your chest to rise and your torso and belly area to expand. Hold this inhale, then slowly exhale through your nose. Count in your head how long it takes to inhale and how long it takes to exhale. Continue doing these slow deep breaths through your nose until the length of your inhale matches the length of your exhale.

After you get the hang of breathing in this controlled manner, you can start to form a slight constriction at the back of your throat as if you were trying to fog up a mirror. This will cause a gentle sound as you inhale and exhale. Don't

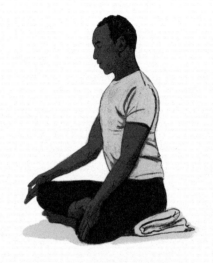

worry if this is inconsistent at first. It takes time and practice to become comfortable with the Ujjayi breath. Just continue to make observations about the breath and keep things slow and steady. To start, practice for 3 to 5 minutes. This is the breath that is used throughout asana practice to create a rhythm in our movements and calm the mind, even in the most challenging moments.

Meditation

Meditation is the stilling of the mind, a break from restless emotions and thoughts. If you're like me and almost everyone I know, your mind rarely sits still. Instead, it runs a constant loop of to-do lists, reflections, plans, and worries. Because of this, we're rarely ever truly *here*. Ram Dass, the American spiritual teacher, revolutionized this concept in the 1970s with his book, *Be Here Now*. He claimed that we're always in the past or future but never actually in the present, and he led millions of people to sit in meditation to experience its powerful effects. Meditation allows us to become an observer of our thoughts and emotions instead of being ruled by them.

STARTER
5-MINUTE MEDITATION

The easiest way to start a meditation practice is to use your breath. Find a quiet space where you can close your eyes and focus for 5 minutes. (It's helpful to set a timer to make sure you don't end earlier or go much longer than you anticipated.)

Sit or lie down in a comfortable position. Close your eyes and draw your attention to your breath. You don't have to do anything; this is simply a time to observe the breath. Focus only on your inhales and exhales for 5 minutes. Whenever your mind wanders away from the breath, bring your focus back to it. There is no right or wrong here. Do your best to continually draw your focus back to the breath and the moment.

2

Preparing for Yoga

Yoga requires dedication and a time commitment. To experience the amazing benefits of yoga, you'll need to prioritize it in your schedule the best you can. Once you do that, choosing the time of day that fits your mood, getting the tools to do your practice, creating a space, and preparing your body for it are the next steps.

You Are Unique

Your body is unique. None of us is created exactly the same. Men and women have different bone structures. You may be dealing with an injury, illness, or changes that come from aging. You may have tightness where everyone else seems to be flexible. This doesn't mean you should limit your yoga practice. Instead, tailor your practice to more fully support your body's needs.

You also have your own unique nature and personality. Adapting your practice to your mental state each day will help you reap the benefits. Certain postures are designed to calm and others to energize. When you come to the mat, check in with yourself. If you are stressed, you may want to do a practice that is calming. Or if you are sluggish, you may want to choose a practice that is energizing.

Adjusting Your Mind

One of the best ways to get yourself ready for a fulfilling yoga practice is to change your mind-set. If you begin with the attitude that you're too busy, too inflexible, or just don't see the point, you're going to have a difficult time incorporating yoga into your life.

Remember that yoga is not a task or goal or even a means of "self-improvement." It's about being in the moment. Yoga isn't meant to change you. Let go of any expectations about the outcome. Instead, approach it with an open mind and total acceptance of the now.

Finding Time

Once your mind is open and you feel ready, find a time to practice yoga every day. Traditionally, yogis practiced around sunrise or sunset because those were viewed as the most calm and serene times of day. Think about the calmest moments of your day. Is this when you first wake up? When the house is quiet in the late evening? When you usually have an afternoon lull? Try to commit to rolling out the mat at this time each day.

If you can't fit in an hour-long practice every day, that's OK. Seek out short chunks of time to sit and breathe throughout the day. These are tiny yoga moments, space to quiet your mind. Giving yourself even a small break from your daily routine is important.

Tools of the Trade

While nothing is required to practice yoga except having a mind and a body, and being able to breathe, there are some tools that will help you in the practice. These tools can be used for asana and meditation.

FOR ASANA

Several simple items can make the physical practice of yoga easier and more adaptable to your own unique body type:

Yoga mat. The mat is key because it prevents slipping and creates a solid footing for your poses. When practicing in large groups, it also becomes your own sacred space. Look for a mat that has a bit of grip to it. You do not want your hands or feet to slide on the mat while holding poses. Mats come in many different colors, thicknesses, and textures. The thinner ones are great for travel. Thicker mats work well for seated, supine, or restorative practices, providing more cushioning on the joints and bones. The rougher mats are stickier, and they are best for Vinyasa (more dynamic) classes. Be sure to stay away from mats made with PVC material, even though they are cheap. I use a natural rubber mat, ⅙ inch thick, and it is great for everything!

Yoga blocks. Blocks can be used to help you adapt the poses to your own body. For example, if your hamstrings are tight, you can use blocks to bring the ground closer to you when bending forward. Look for blocks that are sturdy but not too hard. Blocks come in different heights and materials. I prefer standard cork blocks, which can be used at three different heights. Cork is a natural material of medium firmness—sturdier than foam and more forgiving than wood.

MAKING A COMMITMENT

At first, it may be challenging to hold your commitment. Here are some tips to help you prioritize your practice.

- Place your mat out at night. In the morning it will be a gentle reminder to meditate or begin your practice.
- Schedule your practice as an appointment in your calendar.
- Sign up for a recurring class at your local yoga studio so that you commit to going once or twice per week.
- Set an alarm on your phone. Write a nice message to yourself with that alarm that tells you it's time to for a little "me" time. Don't hit snooze.
- Set a goal to practice once a week for eight weeks, or whatever seems doable for you. When you reach that goal, reward yourself. Buy a new mat or cook your favorite meal. Do something that makes you happy.
- Find a quote or a mantra, or create one of your own. Write it down in your journal, or frame it and place it next to your bed or your yoga space. Let it inspire you to dedicate time to your practice.

Yoga strap. Yoga straps can be used for passive stretching, active poses, and to aid in more advanced postures that require "binding," where the hands are joined behind the back. When looking for a strap, look for one that has a metal closure on the end so that the strap can be made into an adjustable loop.

Bolster. A bolster is great for meditating or sitting or lying down for extended periods of time. Bolsters are rectangular in shape and feel like a firm, sturdy pillow. They're wonderful props for restorative yoga, and make the greatest gift for prenatal yoga. Use them to support all your seated and supine poses for more ease and comfort.

Blanket. Blankets can be used as a prop to help you get into poses, to pad your knees, or to lift your seat. They can also be used for warmth at the end of practice. Most yoga blankets are fairly stiff and durable and can be stacked for varying heights and needs. Many yoga blankets are made from wool, which can be very hot. I prefer woven cotton blankets.

FOR MEDITATION

Meditation only requires the ability to close your eyes and breathe, but a few enhancements can make meditation more comfortable and inviting:

A meditation cushion, bolster, or one or two stacked blankets. In the beginning, your knees and hips may be uncomfortable during seated meditation. Elevating your seat will relieve this discomfort and allow you to sit up tall.

Music. Soft, soothing music that helps drown out outside noise and calm or focus your mind can be a helpful aid to your meditation practice.

Incense. If you start a practice by burning incense every time, it will become an olfactory signal to your body that it's time to meditate.

Aromatherapy oils. These are oils that you apply to the body to create a similar effect as incense. Choose a smell that resonates with you and makes you feel calm.

Prerecorded meditation. If you find it difficult to meditate or calm your active mind, try using a prerecorded meditation. You can easily find these online or on iTunes. Look for a recording that matches the time you want to allot to meditation and search for a voice that is soothing to you.

CLOTHING

Some ads would have you believe you have to run out and buy the latest yoga pants before you even hit the mat. Trendy yoga gear isn't necessary, but you do want to have clothing that's comfortable and allows you to move with ease. Look for tops that are fairly formfitting. You don't want your shirt falling down in your face when you're in Downward-Facing Dog or other inversions. Pants should be made of

Ayurveda means "the science of life" and is one of the great ancient tools to help you discover your physical and emotional tendencies. Ayurveda categorizes our physical, emotional, and mental characteristics into three *doshas*, or mind-body types: *Vata*, *Pitta*, and *Kapha*. Each dosha is characterized by the elements of earth, water, fire, air, and ether.

You can find many online quizzes to discover your specific dosha. By identifying your mind-body type, you can create a lifestyle and yoga practice to support your nature. Practicing yoga for your dosha builds on the philosophy of "like increases like." The idea, therefore, is to add in opposite elements to achieve a balanced state. The following are descriptions of the three doshas, including dominant characteristics and balancing elements, to help give you an idea of your type.

Vata: Air and Ether. A person with a predominant Vata dosha is usually thin with a light frame. They are creative and high-energy, but also a bit spacey and likely to experience sudden bouts of fatigue. They welcome change and new experiences, but when imbalanced can suffer from anxiety and insomnia. A grounding, calming, and warming practice and lifestyle will balance Vata's excess air and ether elements, and reduce their fearful tendencies.

Pitta: Fire and Water. Someone with a dominant Pitta dosha is usually of medium size and weight. They are intellectual and have a strong ability to concentrate, but can also be short-tempered and argumentative. They are sharp-witted and often outspoken with abundant energy, but when imbalanced can suffer from ulcers, excessive body heat, and heartburn. A more cooling and heart-centered practice and lifestyle counteract Pitta's fire. Spending time in nature and by water is nurturing for Pitta as well.

Kapha: Earth and Water. Those with a predominant Kapha dosha are strongly built. They love routine and are naturally calm and thoughtful, but can also be stubborn and resistant to change. They operate in a slow and steady manner, but when imbalanced they may put on extra weight and become at risk for asthma and diabetes. Anything energetic and uplifting balances Kapha's earth and water sluggishness. This constitution benefits greatly from movement.

a material that allows you to move freely, and formfitting enough so they won't fall down when you are lying down and raise your legs in the air.

Clearing Space

Joseph Campbell once said, "Your sacred space is where you can find yourself over and over again." Since yoga is the practice of discovering and honoring your true self, it's important to create a regular space in your home or office to practice yoga.

Choose somewhere that can be a refuge from the distractions of the outside world. Look for a place where you can find quiet, but also move easily. Then equip your space with the essentials of your practice: a mat, props, candle, or anything else that makes it comfortable and special. Add one thing that serves as a reminder that it's

SPECIAL CONDITIONS

Some special conditions may affect your practice. It's best to be aware of these in advance.

Pregnancy. When pregnant, you'll need to make adjustments for your changing body and shifting center of gravity. Practice open twists, to make room for your growing belly, instead of deep twists, such as Seated Spinal Twist (page 165), that constrict the belly while pregnant. Also avoid lying down on your belly for backbends such as Locust Pose (page 145) while pregnant. Always tell your teacher that you're pregnant before class begins so they can recommend modifications.

Menstruation. Traditionally women who were in what is called their "moon cycle" were told not to practice inversions, but this has been largely dismissed in modern yoga. I suggest calling on your intuition during menstruation. If you're having pain or discomfort, more restorative yoga would be best. If you're sluggish, inversions could actually be just the cure to lift your energy and mood! During this time, it is important to listen to your body.

Injury. If you have a serious injury, consult with your doctor before beginning an asana practice. Also, listen to your body. The idea of "no pain, no gain" doesn't exist in yoga. When you are injured is not the time to push your body to its limits. Be gentle to your body and let it heal.

a sacred space, such as a photo, a passage from a book, a framed quote, a trinket from a trip, or a gift from someone special. You will want to have a timer to use with meditation.

Priming Your Body

One of the best ways to prepare your body for yoga is through nutrition. Good nutrition complements a yoga practice by giving your body the fuel it needs to perform the tasks at hand. By making better choices with food, you begin to learn to honor your body's needs.

It is best not to eat for two hours before practicing asana. You want your body to be free to move and twist without the added work of having to digest a heavy meal.

Some days you may have aches or pains or feel ill and tired. It is best to adjust your practice accordingly. If the aches or pains do not stem from a serious injury, then you can find poses to ease the pain by stretching the area or relieving a related area. If you feel ill or tired, opt for a more grounding set of poses that involve less movement and more stretching and relaxing.

3

THREE
Asana Practice

"The body is my temple, asanas are my prayers." —B. K. S. IYENGAR

As described in the first chapter, "yoga" means to yoke, or join. In the physical practice of yoga, we use our bodies to join with our spirit.

Ancient yogis realized how difficult it was to calm the mind, and sought a path to liberation. Ultimately they created the asanas that, along with the breath and awareness, helped bring the mind into focus. Thousands of years later, modern yogis bear witness to these teachings.

In the *Yoga Sutras*, "asana" is described as a steady and comfortable seat. Cultivating this grounded energy on our mat and out in the world is the magic formula that creates peace. Asana is the true essence of yoga.

The most important part of your yoga practice is not standing on your head. It's not touching your toes. *It's simply getting on the mat.*

Just the act of committing to your practice—whether you have 10 minutes or an hour—will impact your life. As the great yogic text, the *Bhagavad Gita*, reminds us: "On this path no effort is wasted, no gain is ever reversed; even a little of this practice will shelter you from great sorrow."

Listening to Your Body

In yoga, the breath is coordinated with movement to become a moving meditation, or vinyasa. All movement is guided by smooth and regulated inhalation, retention, exhalation, and the intention to focus the mind and energize the body with prana, or life force.

If your breath becomes choppy, rest in Child's Pose (page 35), return to your rhythmic breath, and then resume movement. All poses and sequences are labeled after the three main healing qualities of nature: energizing, grounding, and calming. Build your practice to best suit the needs of your body and mind.

Remember, this is your practice. Listen to your body and be present, conscious, aware, and mindful of what it tells you. For the sequences in this book, one pose generally flows into the next. I will guide you on how many breaths to take, but you may decide to stay longer or shorter in certain poses. This is how you develop your personal practice.

Approaching Challenging Poses

One of yoga's greatest gifts is the process of working with challenging asanas. In your practice, there will be asanas that you love, and approach with ease and joy each time. You'll also quickly discover asanas that are more of a struggle, and that you want to skip entirely. This, of course, is a mirror for the obstacles and challenges we meet in life and how we choose to react to them.

The key is to approach difficult asanas with compassion and curiosity. The best way to do this is to breathe through the discomfort toward your edge, without forcing yourself into the pose. Remember, a key tenet of yoga is ahimsa, or nonviolence, which also refers to the relationship you have with yourself on the mat. Rather than pushing a pose, back off. Reach for a prop to create more stability or space in the body, or take Child's Pose (page 35) to avoid any strain or stress. Let go.

If you're nursing an injury, consult your physician or physical therapist before you begin practicing yoga. Once you're cleared to practice, honor your injury with proper alignment, patience, and awareness. Back off from any pain or strain. Like challenging poses, injuries are an opportunity to listen to your body rather than your ego and let go of any expectations.

Revolved Half Moon with a Block. A block can aid in alignment, making the asana more attainable and enjoyable.

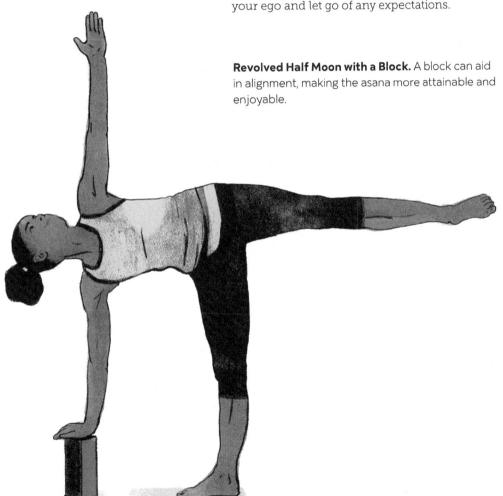

BASIC POSES

Practicing the asanas is how you'll build your yoga practice. It's best to start with the basics. These asanas are included in most yoga sequences and are part of a well-rounded yoga practice.

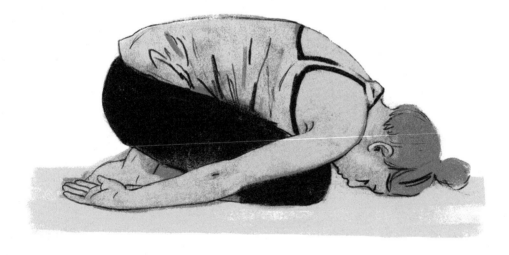

Child's Pose

Balasana

This pose is called Child's Pose because it will help you develop a beginner's mind. This pose soothes the whole nervous system and calms the mind. You can return to it any time you need a break during a session. It's also a great way to start your practice.

QUALITY Grounding   **EFFECT** Tranquility   **PROPS** Blanket under the knees (optional)   **GAZE** Internal

1 Come on to your hands and knees. Send your hips back toward your heels, laying your chest on the tops of your thighs. Stretch your arms forward and rest your head on the ground with your eyes closed. Another variation is to stretch your arms back by your sides and release your hands by your heels for a deeper restorative experience.

2 Take 5 long, deep breaths, slowing down to a 4-count inhale and a 4-count exhale. With each exhale, send your sit bones down toward your heels to release the lower back.

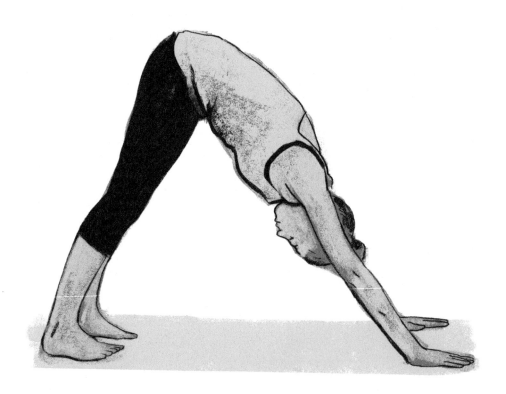

Downward-Facing Dog Pose

Adho Mukha Svanasana

This pose honors man's best friend and its natural stretching pose. Downward-Facing Dog lengthens the back of the legs and spine while strengthening the arms and legs and cleansing and nourishing the brain with blood and oxygen.

QUALITY Grounding   **EFFECT** Flexibility, strength   **PROPS** None   **GAZE** Between the feet

1   Come on to your hands and knees with your hands directly under your shoulders and with your knees under your hips. Root down through your thumb and index finger as you roll your shoulders back and away from your ears. Tuck your toes under and lift your hips to the sky as you lengthen your legs behind you and draw your heels toward the ground.

2   Bend your knees slightly. Draw your chest toward your thighs to stretch open your shoulders and lengthen your neck. Then slowly straighten your legs again as you continue to press your hands into the ground, and release (relax) your head between your arms.

3   Keep your gaze between your feet. Take 5 deep breaths. As you exhale, push your heels closer to the ground. Release into Child's Pose (page 35).

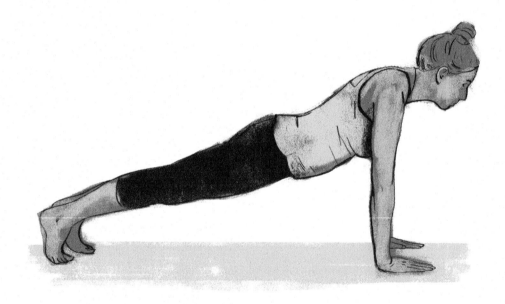

Plank Pose

Utthita Chaturanga Dandasana

Plank pose is a simple beginner's pose that strengthens your body and prepares you for some of the more challenging poses such as arm balances and inversions.

QUALITY Energizing **EFFECT** Heat, strength **PROPS** None **GAZE** Forward

1 Begin on your hands and knees with your hands directly under your shoulders and your fingers spread wide. Lengthen your right leg straight back behind you with your toes tucked under. When you feel stable, lengthen the left leg to join the right, toes tucked under.

2 Flex your feet by reaching both heels back strongly and engaging your thighs. Reach forward with your chest and draw your shoulders back away from your ears.

3 Lift your navel and the sides of your abdomen in and up, along with lifting the ribs.

4 Lift your head so it's in line with your spine, and look forward.

5 Stay in this position for 5 breaths before releasing into Child's Pose (page 35).

A

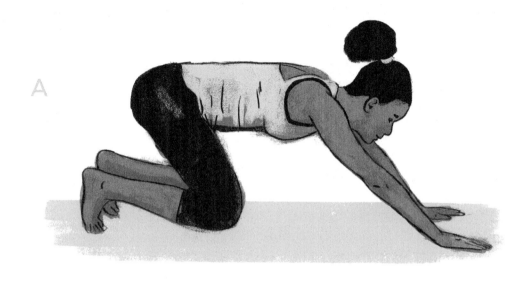

B

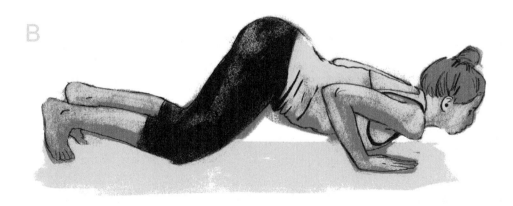

Knees, Chest, Chin Pose

Ashtanga Namaskara

A great pose to prepare for challenging arm balances, this pose strengthens the arms and opens the chest. It's a transition pose into Baby Cobra (page 45) in Full Sun Salutation (page 199).

QUALITY Grounding   **EFFECT** Strength   **PROPS** None   **GAZE** Forward

1 Begin in Plank Pose (page 39). Release your knees to the ground (A) followed by your chest and chin by bending your elbows by your side close to your ribs (B).

2 Lift your shoulders off the ground by pressing your hands into the ground and drawing your elbows in.

3 Release your pelvis to the ground to rise up into Baby Cobra or send your hips back to your heels into Child's Pose (page 35).

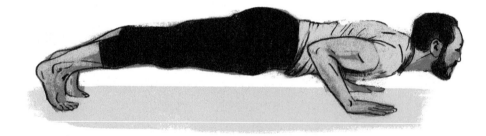

Yogi's Push-Up Pose

Chaturanga Dandasana

In Sanskrit, chaturanga means "four-limbed staff pose." This is basically a push-up with your elbows tucked in. This pose strengthens you inside and out, and is an integral part of the Full Sun Salutation series (page 199).

QUALITY Energizing **EFFECT** Strength **PROPS** None **GAZE** Forward

1 Begin in Plank Pose (page 39). Reach your heels back to activate your legs, and reach forward with your chest by drawing your shoulders up and away from your ears.

2 Lift your ribs and navel up and draw your tailbone in to support your lower back.

3 Bend your elbows by your sides and lower down to about 3 inches from the ground while continuing to lift your navel and front body. This is a challenging pose. Hold for 1 to 3 breaths, or for as long as you can, with your gaze about 6 inches in front of you. Then drop down or move into Baby Cobra (page 45) or Upward-Facing Dog (page 47).

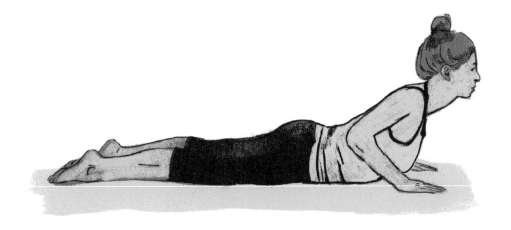

Baby Cobra Pose

Bhujangasana

This pose is a simple backbend that opens the chest and shoulders while strengthening and toning the upper back and buttocks. It's part of the Full Sun Salutation series (page 199), but can also be practiced alone.

QUALITY Energizing **EFFECT** Openness, strength **PROPS** None **GAZE** Up

1 Begin by lying facedown on the ground. Draw your legs together. Bend your elbows and place your hands by your upper ribs. Draw your elbows toward each other to lift the shoulders. Press strongly into your hands to lift your head, shoulders, and chest off the ground as you inhale.

2 Keep your chin slightly down to lengthen the back of your neck. Turn your gaze upward between your eyebrows.

3 Stay for about 3 breaths, pressing your weight into your hands and the tops of your feet.

4 Lower your head down and press back into a Child's Pose (page 35) or Downward-Facing Dog (page 37).

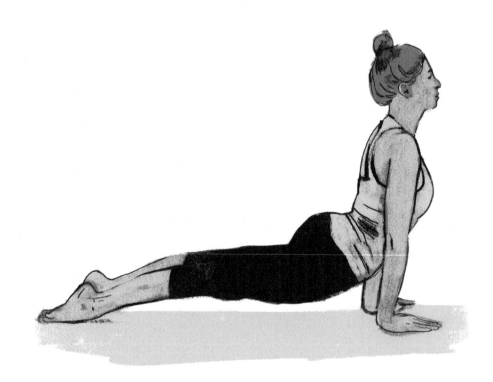

Upward-Facing Dog Pose

Urdhva Mukha Svanasana

Another wonderful pose inspired by our canine friends, this is a more challenging version of Baby Cobra (page 45). It's a powerful and invigorating pose that releases blocked energy.

QUALITY Energizing   EFFECT Openness, strength   PROPS Blocks   GAZE Forward and slightly up

1   Begin by lying facedown on the ground. Bend your elbows and slide your hands down so they're in line with your bottom ribs. Press down into your hands and the tops of your feet and straighten your arms, lifting your head, chest, abdomen, pelvis, and thighs off the ground.

2   Draw your shoulders away from your ears as you press down through your thumbs and index fingers. Move your chest forward and up between your arms, and press your pelvis down to lengthen your spine. Lower your chin slightly to protect your neck as you take your gaze up.

3   This is an intense pose, so take 1 to 5 breaths before slowly exhaling back into Downward-Facing Dog (page 37) or Child's Pose (page 35). If you don't yet have the flexibility to accomplish this pose as described, you can place blocks under your hands to bring the ground to you.

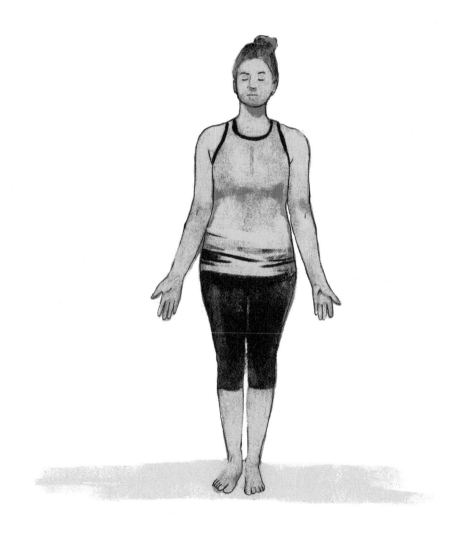

Mountain Pose

Tadasana

This pose seems so simple, but to stand still, tall, strong, and present can be challenging. As the name suggests, Mountain Pose increases strength, confidence, and stability. It also helps with body awareness—like you're seeing it all from the mountaintop.

QUALITY Grounding   **EFFECT** Focus, stability, strength   **PROPS** None   **GAZE** Forward

1 Begin by standing up tall with your feet hip-distance apart and your arms by your sides. Widen your heels a tiny bit. Draw your tailbone down and navel back to lengthen your lower back.

2 Draw your shoulders back and down to open and lift your chest as you draw your lower ribs in.

3 Keep your head reaching up as you slightly draw your chin in toward your throat to lengthen the back of your neck. Release your jaw and keep your eyes soft with your gaze forward.

4 Take 5 breaths here, exhaling your feet in to the earth to feel rooted, and inhaling your head high to feel elevated, like a mountain!

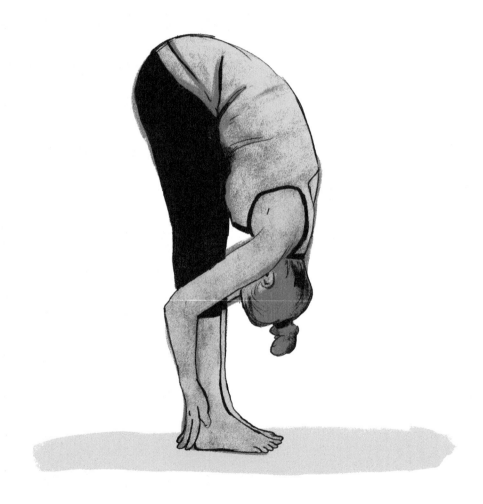

Standing Forward Bend Pose

Uttanasana

This pose calms and soothes the mind while releasing tension from the back and spine and increasing flexibility in the backs of the legs. It also tones the internal organs through a slight compression, promoting digestion.

QUALITY Calming **EFFECT** Cleansing, flexibility **PROPS** Blocks **GAZE** Internal

1 Start in Mountain Pose (page 49). Inhale your arms up and exhale to fold forward over your legs, hinging at the hips. Bend your knees as much as you need to to lay your chest on your thighs. Place your hands on the ground or on blocks.

2 Shift slightly forward to evenly distribute your weight on your feet. Lift the front of your thighs as you stretch the backs of your legs.

3 Keep a slight bend in the knees to avoid hyperextending them. Keep your thighs engaged while completely releasing your spine and softening your belly, face, and jaw.

4 Inhale to lift the chest slightly away from the legs and exhale to release into the pose a bit deeper. Stay here for 3 to 5 breaths.

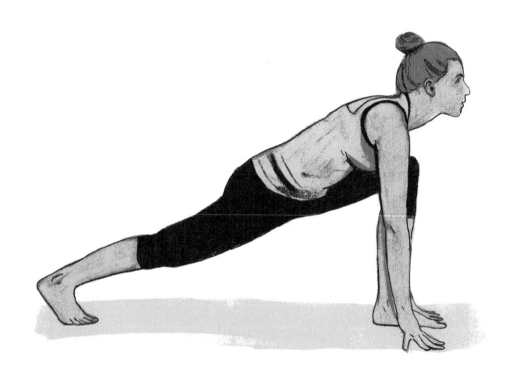

Low Lunge Pose

Anjaneyasana

This basic standing pose is a core asana in the Full Sun Salutation series (page 199) and is also frequently used as a transition pose in sequences. It has many variations. All of them simultaneously build strength and flexibility.

QUALITY Grounding   **EFFECT** Strength, flexibility   **PROPS** Blocks   **GAZE** Forward

1 Begin in Mountain Pose (page 49) and fold forward into a Standing Forward Bend (page 51) as you exhale. As you inhale, reach your left leg back behind you into a low lunge (pictured), with your right knee between your hands. Stay directly over your right ankle as you stretch back through your left heel and flex your left toes. You can place blocks under your hands to help lift your chest.

2 Release your hips down and lift your left thigh as you stretch your chest forward, drawing your shoulders back. Lift your head in line with your spine and gaze forward. Stay for 3 breaths, exhaling deeper into the pose with each breath.

3 Step forward with the left leg. Repeat on the other side by stepping back with the right leg.

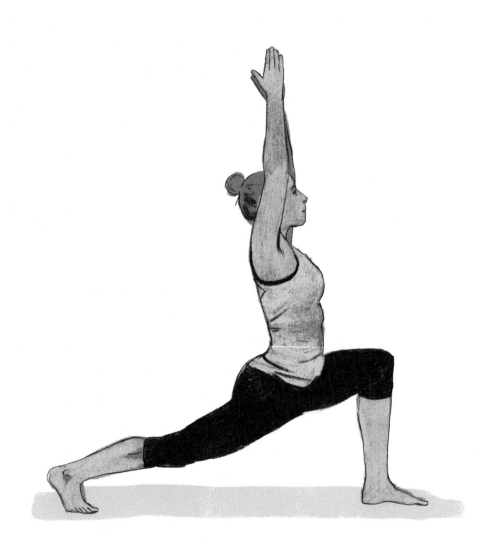

High Lunge Pose

Utthita Ashwa Sanchalanasana

High Lunge increases strength in the thighs and back body, or back side of the body. It also opens the groin and hip flexors.

QUALITY Grounding, energizing   EFFECT Flexibility, strength   PROPS None
GAZE Forward and slightly up

1 Follow all the steps for Low Lunge (page 53). Then reach your arms forward and up as your hips continue to drop down. Reach up to the sky.

2 Bend your left knee a little to allow your hips to release down and to lengthen your lower back and stretch your left hip flexor.

3 Lift your rib cage, soften your lower ribs in, and reach up actively with your arms. Draw your shoulders down and away from your ears to lengthen your neck.

4 Keep your gaze steady and forward and take 3 breaths. Reach up higher with each inhale, and sink your hips downward as you continue to reach the inner left thigh up.

5 Step forward with the left leg. Repeat on the other side by stepping back with the right leg.

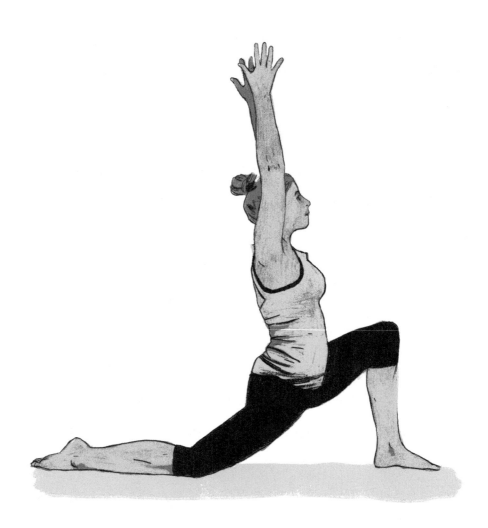

Crescent Moon Pose

Anjaneyasana

Crescent Moon is a deep lunge that's a great way to prepare your body for backbends. The pose is energizing and grounding. It also increases flexibility in the spine and quadriceps and opens up the hip flexors.

QUALITY Grounding, energizing   **EFFECT** Flexibility   **PROPS** Blanket   **GAZE** Forward and up

1   Follow the steps for Low Lunge (page 53), but release the left knee to the ground. You can place a folded blanket down to protect your knee.

2   Reach your arms up as you do in High Lunge (page 55), but reach back into a backbend.

3   Make sure to draw your tailbone down as the pubis lifts to protect your lower back. Draw your lower belly back to protect the sacral spine.

4   Take 3 breaths in the pose, releasing deeper with each exhale.

5   Step forward with the left leg. Repeat on the other side by stepping back with the right leg.

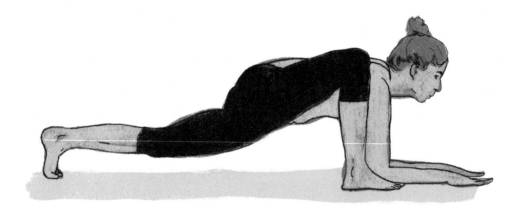

Lizard Lunge Pose

Utthan Pristhasana

This lunge is a deep hip stretch and is a great way to prepare for more advanced hip openers. It also strengthens and stretches the thighs, knees, and chest.

QUALITY Grounding, calming   **EFFECT** Flexibility   **PROPS** Blocks   **GAZE** Forward and down

1 Make your way into Downward-Facing Dog (page 37). As you inhale, raise your right leg, bend your knee, and reach your right heel toward your left sit bone to open up your hip. As you exhale, step your right foot up to the outside of your right hand and walk your right foot to the right edge of your mat. If the stretch is too intense, come onto your fingertips. For a deep hip stretch, place blocks under your hands and open your knee to the right while grounding down into your right big toe.

2 Sink down into your hips as you lift your chest and gaze forward. Release your back knee down, if needed. Release your forearms to the ground for an even deeper hip stretch.

3 Stay in the pose for 3 breaths, deepening the stretch with each exhale.

4 Step forward with the left leg. Repeat with the right leg.

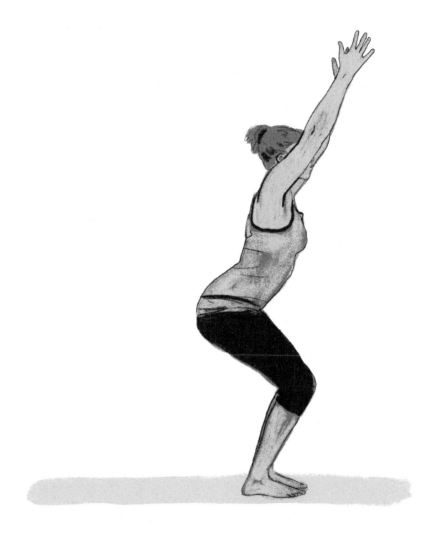

Powerful Pose

Utkatasana

As the name suggests, this pose builds inner power, strength, and heat by drawing all your energy inside your body. With the longer hold, it fires up your legs and abdominal muscles—as well as your willpower. This pose is also called Lightning Bolt because of both its shape and energizing quality!

QUALITY Energizing   **EFFECT** Heat, strength   **PROPS** None   **GAZE** Forward and up

1 Begin in Mountain Pose (page 49). Inhale your arms up and exhale to bend your knees as you send your hips back and down so your thighs are parallel to the ground.

2 Keep sinking down while drawing your tailbone down and lifting the navel back to lengthen your lower back.

3 Lift your chest but soften your lower ribs down to avoid overarching. Draw your shoulders down and away from your ears as you reach your arms up or join them as if in prayer.

4 Look forward. Keep the back of your neck long by slightly releasing your chin and jaw.

5 Stay for 5 steady breaths before coming up to stand in Mountain Pose with your arms by your sides.

STANDING POSES

Standing poses are full-body poses and the core of any yoga practice. They cultivate strength and flexibility simultaneously, not one at the expense of the other. They heat the body for improved digestion and bring flexibility to the hips, legs, feet, arms, chest, shoulders, and spine, all the while making deeper poses possible through repetition. They can be practiced on their own or as a part of a sequence. Make sure to always practice standing poses on the right side first, and then the left side, allowing for consistency and a natural clockwise movement.

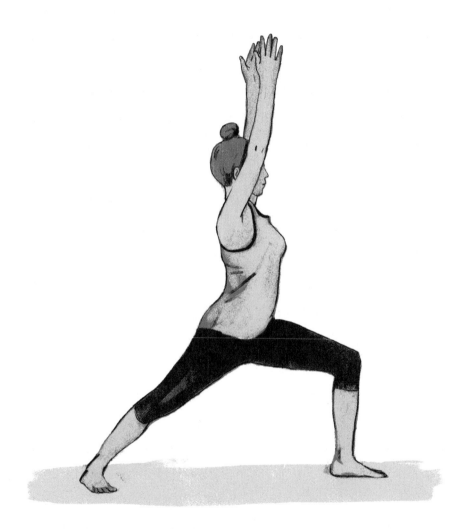

Warrior I Pose

Virabhadrasana I

This pose awakens the inner warrior, arousing strength and courage to face the day and others with compassion. It strengthens the back of the body and legs while opening the chest, heart, and lungs for increased energy and stamina. It also cultivates deep focus.

QUALITY Grounding   **EFFECT** Balance, energy, strength   **PROPS** None   **GAZE** Forward and up

1 Begin in Downward-Facing Dog (page 37). Reach your right leg up to the sky and exhale, placing it between your hands into a Low Lunge (page 53). Release your left heel into the ground by turning it in slightly so your whole foot is on the ground.

2 Inhale your arms and torso forward and up, vertical to the ground.

3 Keep drawing your right hip back and left hip forward as you reach your left leg back. Root down the outer edge of your left foot by lifting your arch.

4 Sink down through your hips as you reach up with your spine, arms, and gaze. If you can, join your palms together while drawing your shoulders down and away from your ears, and soften the front ribs to lengthen the lower back.

5 Stay for 3 to 5 breaths and return to Downward-Facing Dog to repeat on the left side.

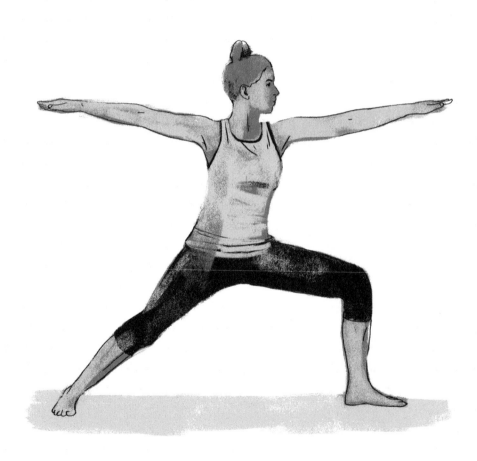

Warrior II Pose

Virabhadrasana II

This pose is like a brave warrior: beautiful and strong. It increases flexibility in the hips, shoulders, chest, and arms while building strength in the legs and knees and encouraging deep focus and will.

QUALITY Grounding, energizing   **EFFECT** Flexibility, strength   **PROPS** None   **GAZE** Forward

1 Standing in the middle of your mat, begin in Mountain Pose (page 49) with your hands at the center of your heart as if in prayer.

2 Step or jump your feet and arms out to the sides with your feet directly under your hands. As you inhale, reach your arms up and turn your right leg out, facing the front of your mat. Turn your left foot in at a 45-degree angle. As you exhale, bend your right knee directly over your right ankle. Release your arms to be parallel with the ground and gaze over your right hand.

3 Track your right knee toward your pinky toe and sink deeply into your hips, making sure your knee does not go past your ankle.

4 Draw your tailbone down as your pubic bone lifts. Draw your belly up and back as your bottom ribs draw in.

5 Relax your shoulders down and away from your ears to lengthen the back of your neck. Draw your shoulder blades together to open your chest.

6 Keep your gaze focused and steady over your right hand. With your fingers together, reach your hands forward and back at the same time to symbolize the past behind you, the future in front of you, and you present in the moment.

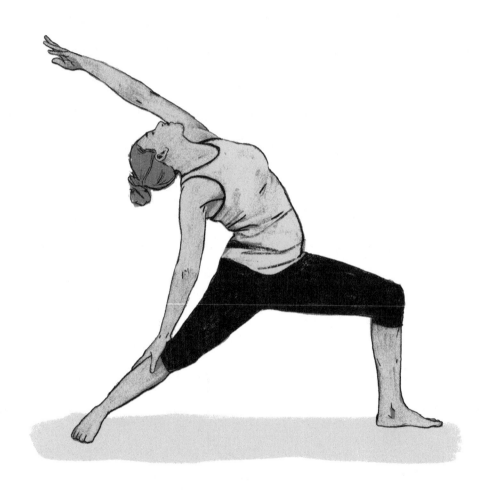

Peaceful Warrior Pose

Virabhadrasana Shanti

This posture honors all of the peaceful warriors and spiritual activists out there. It builds strength in the legs and stretches the side body, opening the heart.

QUALITY Grounding, energizing   **EFFECT** Flexibility, openness, strength   **PROPS** None   **GAZE** Up

1 Begin in Warrior II (page 67). As you inhale, tip backward and lift your right arm over your head, looking up. Slide your left hand down your left leg, draw your left hip forward a bit, and arch back.

2 Stay here for 1 to 3 breaths before returning to Warrior II, and switch to the other side.

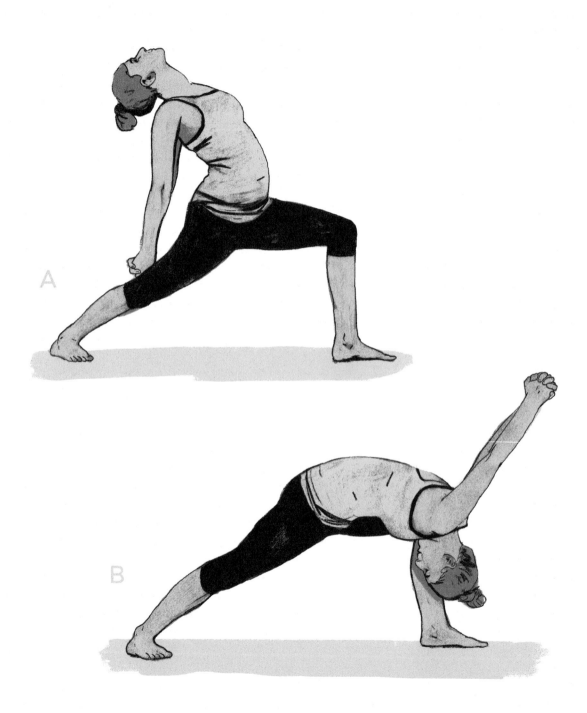

Humble Warrior Pose

Virabhadrasana Bhakti

We may not think of "humble" and "warrior" going together, but this pose honors the courage it takes to surrender. It opens the hips and shoulders and stretches the spine as well as clearing and calming the mind.

QUALITY Grounding   **EFFECT** Flexibility, strength   **PROPS** Strap   **GAZE** Inward

1 Begin in Warrior I (page 65) with your right leg forward. Release your arms by your sides and interlace your fingers behind your back. Stretch open your chest and inhale (A). As you exhale, bow your head toward the ground on the inside of your right leg (B).

2 Inhale to rise back up to Warrior I, and exhale into Downward-Facing Dog (page 37) to switch sides.

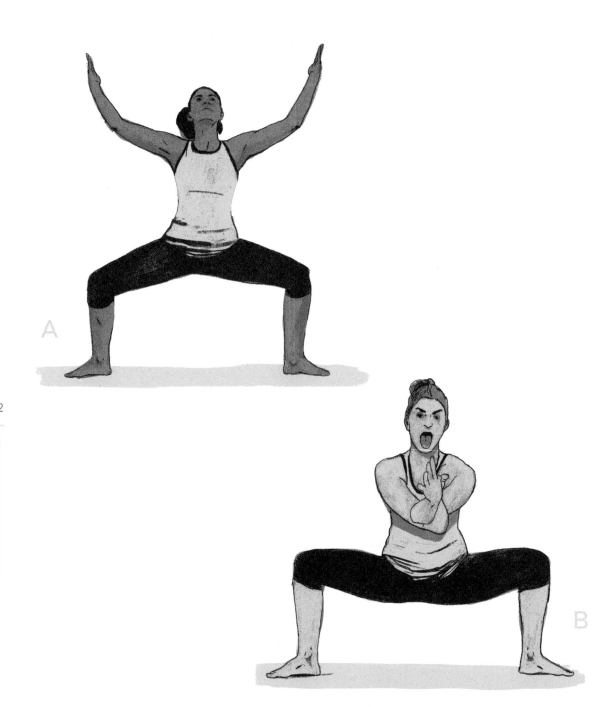

Warrior Goddess Pose

Shakti Asana

This goddess pose is fierce and fiery and will make you feel the burn. It opens the hips and strengthens the thighs and buttocks. Be mindful of your knees in this pose—always make sure they are directly over your ankles, not in front of your ankles.

QUALITY Grounding, energizing **EFFECT** Flexibility, heat, strength **PROPS** None **GAZE** Forward

1 Come to the center of your mat and step or hop your feet wide out to the sides. Turn your toes out and inhale your arms up above your head. As you exhale, bend your knees over your ankles and lift your arms into a cactus shape, with your elbows in line with your shoulders and your forearms vertical to the ground (A).

2 Elongate your tailbone toward the ground and lift up through your navel as you continue to sink down.

3 Draw your thighbones in toward your hips as your knees reach outward. Stay here for 5 breaths.

4 On the last breath, hook your right arm under the left into the upper half of the Eagle Pose (page 105) and exhale a Lion's Breath three times. Lion's Breath is a purifying breath: Inhale through your nose and exhale powerfully through your mouth as you stick out your tongue and even roar (B).

5 Inhale your arms up, straighten your legs, and hop your feet together into Mountain Pose (page 49).

OPEN STANDING POSES

Open standing poses are awesome asanas that energize, stretch, and strengthen the whole body and make all the more advanced poses possible. Be sure to spend a lot of time in these positions as part of your regular practice.

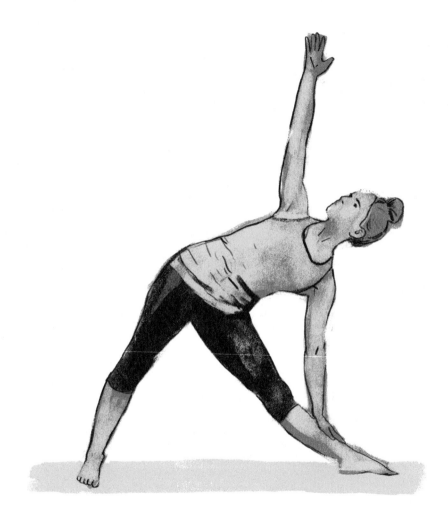

Triangle Pose

Trikonasana

Triangle Pose stretches the hamstrings and hips and opens the chest and shoulders. It reduces stress and anxiety and creates mental stability and balance. This popular pose strengthens the legs, back, and neck and helps with sciatica.

QUALITY Balancing   **EFFECT** Flexibility, stability, strength   **PROPS** Block   **GAZE** Up

1 Begin standing at the top of your mat with your feet hip-distance apart and your arms at your sides.

2 Step or hop your feet wide apart, about 4 to 5 feet.

3 Turn your right foot out 90 degrees so your toes are pointing to the top of the mat. Center your right knee over your right ankle. Pivot your left foot slightly inward so your back toes are at a 45-degree angle.

4 Inhale and raise your arms out to the sides in line with your shoulders, so they're parallel to the ground and aligned directly over your legs. With your palms facing down, reach actively from fingertip to fingertip.

5 As you inhale, reach forward with your right hand and draw your left hip back. Deepen the crease of your right hip and release your right hand down to your shin or a block placed behind your right shin. Turn your left palm forward, with your fingertips reaching toward the sky, and twist your chest open toward the sky. Soften your left hip down slightly.

6 Gently turn your head to gaze up at your right hand. Draw your chin in toward your throat to lengthen the back of your neck.

7 Stay and breathe for up to 5 breaths, opening the chest on each inhale and drawing your ribs and navel in on each exhale.

8 Inhale to stand and repeat on the other side.

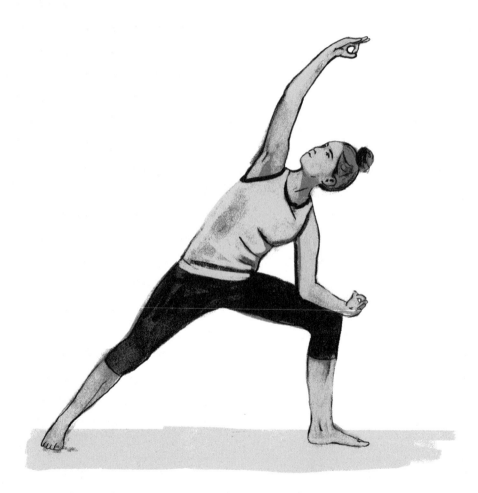

Extended Side Angle Pose

Utthita Parsvakonasana

This wonderful full-body pose includes an intense side stretch. It's energizing and relieves blocked energy from the hips and chest, also strengthening and toning the legs and back.

QUALITY Grounding **EFFECT** Flexibility, strength **PROPS** Block **GAZE** Up

1 Begin in Warrior II (page 67) on the right side. Place your right forearm on your right thigh with your hand facing up and stretch your left arm up over your head. Turn your gaze up toward your left hand and stay for 5 breaths.

2 Press actively through the outside edge of your left foot as you lift the arch. Ground down into the earth as you reach away in the opposite direction.

3 Draw the pelvis forward as you press your left thigh back and open your right knee toward the pinky toe of your right foot.

4 Soften your left hip down and twist your torso open toward the sky, drawing your shoulders back to open your chest.

5 Keep your chin slightly in toward your throat to lengthen and protect your neck as you look up.

6 Inhale up to Warrior II. Straighten your legs and switch sides.

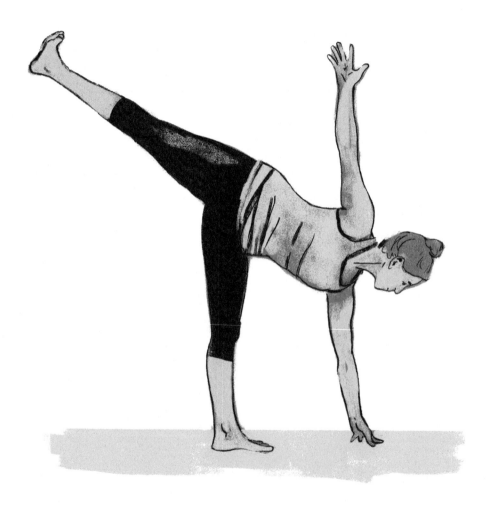

Half Moon Pose

Ardha Chandrasana

One of the most beautiful poses in yoga, Half Moon honors the phases of the moon and celebrates the dark and the light. It creates balance in the body and mind and in your life. The pose strengthens the back body and standing leg, while opening and stretching the top leg and front body. As a transition pose in many sequences, it brings about grace and coordination.

QUALITY Balancing   **EFFECT** Flexibility, focus, strength   **PROPS** Block
GAZE To the ground for stability or to the top hand for energy

1   Begin in Warrior II (page 67) on the right side. Place your left hand on your left hip and stretch your right arm forward as you draw your right hip back.

2   Place your right hand on the ground or on a block 6 inches in front of you and a few inches to the right side of your mat. A block is a great tool when starting out with this pose. Begin shifting your weight forward onto your right hand and foot.

3   Lift up your left leg so it's parallel to the ground and in line with your hips. Lift your left arm up toward the sky, in line with your right arm.

4   Look down at the ground to establish your balance. When you're ready, turn your gaze up toward your left hand and lean back slightly.

5   Flex your left foot and turn your right hip open to stack the hips.

6   Stay here and breathe for 3 to 5 breaths, inhaling to open the front of your body into the light and exhaling the ribs and navel in to open the back body, the shadow side.

7   When you're ready to come down, turn your gaze back to the ground. Bend your right knee while stretching your left leg back and down to the ground. Return to Warrior II before straightening your legs and repeating on the left side.

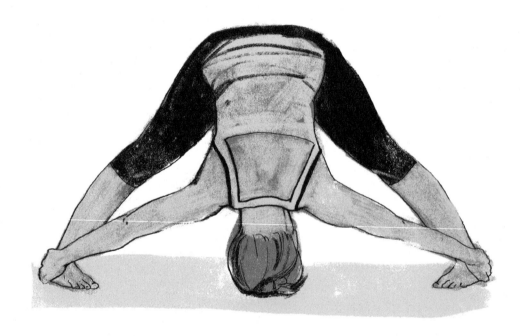

Wide-Legged Forward Bend

Prasarita Padottanasana

This pose is an excellent one to do when you're stressed, tired, or anxious. It's an inversion prep, which calms the mind. Also an invigorating standing pose, it stretches the hamstrings and hips and releases the spine and shoulders.

QUALITY Grounding, calming, energizing   EFFECT Flexibility, strength   PROPS Block   GAZE Forward

1   Begin in Mountain Pose (page 49) and step or hop your feet wide apart, about 4 to 5 feet. Make your feet parallel with the edges of your mat and turn your toes in slightly. Inhale your arms up above your head and exhale to hinge forward at your hips, releasing your hands and head toward the ground.

2   Roll to the outside edges of your feet and lift your arches and inner ankles to energize your inner thighs. If your hamstrings are tight or you're hyperextending or overstretching the backs of your knees, bend your knees slightly to release the spine.

3   Reach for the outer edges of your feet with your hands. Draw your shoulders away from your ears toward your shoulder blades as you release your head closer to the ground. You can place a block or two under your head for support. Stay for 3 to 5 breaths.

VARIATION:

1   For a deeper shoulder stretch, interlace your hands behind your back and exhale your arms closer to the ground in front of you as you draw your palms together.

2   Slowly rise up to stand, bringing your head up last to avoid getting light-headed.

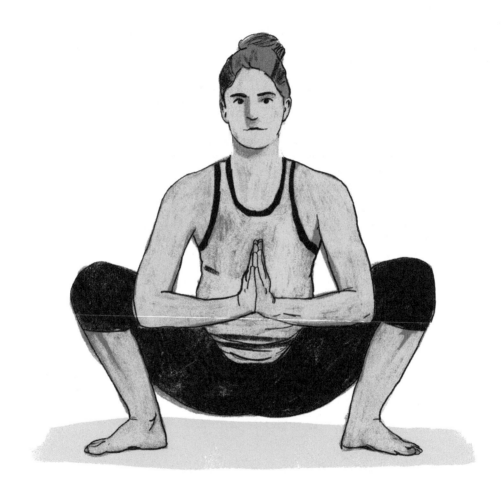

Garland Pose

Malasana

As Westerners, we lose so much mobility in our hips and knees by sitting in chairs for hours on end. This pose reclaims our natural mobility and closeness to the earth by opening the hips and stretching the knees, thighs, groins, and ankle joints, plus lengthening and strengthening the spine. It has also been known to promote elimination and fertility by energizing the organs, and is great preparation for sitting in meditation.

QUALITY Grounding **EFFECT** Flexibility, stability **PROPS** Block **GAZE** Forward and down

1 Begin in Mountain Pose (page 49) with your feet about hip-distance apart. Inhale your arms up above your head and exhale to fold over your legs, hinging at the hips into a Standing Forward Bend (page 51). Bend your knees deeply and lower your hips toward the earth between your heels, turning out your feet slightly.

2 Draw your hands together as if in prayer, with your elbows pressing your knees apart as you widen your thighs. If this is uncomfortable in your knees or ankles, place a block under your sit bones.

3 Exhale to release your hips, and inhale to lengthen your spine and widen your chest by drawing your shoulders down and away from your ears.

4 Soften your chin down slightly to lengthen the back of your neck. Gaze forward and down toward the earth to connect you to the moment.

5 When you're ready, place your hands down on the ground and lengthen your legs into a Standing Forward Bend before you roll back up, vertebra by vertebra, into Mountain Pose.

REVOLVED STANDING POSES

The revolved standing poses are more challenging, intense, fiery, and cleansing than their open standing pose siblings. Practice these poses with the intention of finding peace even within the most challenging situations, and sticking with something no matter how intense it gets. The rewards on the other side are endless.

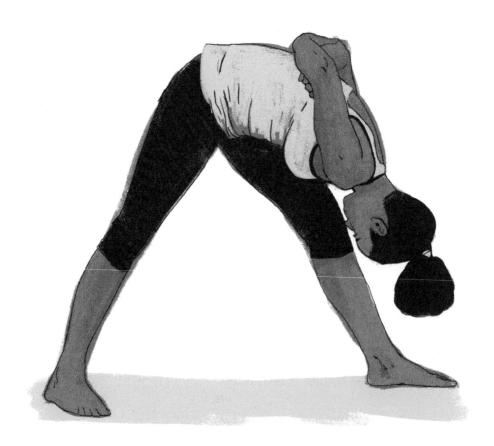

Pyramid Pose

Parsvottanasana

As the name suggests, this pose creates the sacred geometry of a pyramid. It brings about perfect balance and is excellent for stretching the hamstrings and spine, as well as toning and cleansing the internal organs. It's also incredibly calming and rejuvenating for the mind because it sends fresh blood to the brain.

QUALITY Grounding, calming, balancing   EFFECT Flexibility, strength   PROPS Blocks
GAZE Down to the ground

1   Begin in Mountain Pose (page 49) with your feet hip-distance apart. Step your left foot behind you about 3 to 4 feet and release your left heel to the ground. Adjust your feet so the heels of your front and back feet are aligned.

2   Inhale your arms above your head. As you exhale, draw your palms together behind your back in a prayer-like position with your fingers pointing up between your shoulder blades. If a reverse prayer behind your back is too intense, hold on to your opposite elbows.

3   As you inhale, widen your elbows to the side like wings by drawing your shoulders back to stretch open your chest. Arch your back and look up. As you exhale, draw your right hip back and hinge forward at the hips, twisting a bit toward the right. Allow your torso, chest, and head to relax and lengthen over your right leg. Stay here and breathe for 5 breaths.

4   Keep drawing the shoulders back. Lift up as you inhale and exhale deeply from the belly, releasing the spine, head, and jaw.

5   When you're ready to come up, exhale and root down into your feet by shifting your weight back, and inhale to rise up to standing, circling your arms above you. Exhale your left foot forward to meet your right and release your arms by your sides into Mountain Pose. Switch feet and repeat on the other side.

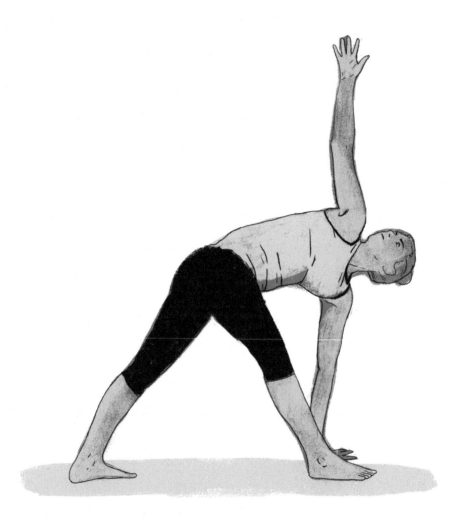

Revolved Triangle Pose

Parivrtta Trikonasana

This pose is a great one to try when you need to spice up your practice. It's heating, cleansing, and invigorating. Make sure your hamstrings, spine, and shoulders are nicely warmed up before you start, and that you have a block nearby.

QUALITY Grounding, energizing   **EFFECT** Cleansing, flexibility, heat, strength
PROPS Block   **GAZE** Up

1   Begin in Mountain Pose (page 49) with your feet hip-distance apart. Step your left foot behind you about 3 to 4 feet and release your left heel to the ground. Adjust your feet as needed so the heels of your front and back feet are aligned.

2   Place your right hand on your right hip and inhale to lift your left arm to the sky. Draw your right hip back as you reach forward with your left hand. Twist over and down toward your right foot. Place a block on the outside of your right foot and adjust it to any height you need, then place your left hand flat on the block. (If this is too uncomfortable, move the block to the inside of your right foot instead.)

3   Rotate your chest and torso to the right, opening your right shoulder toward the sky as you draw your right hip back. Reach your right arm straight up in line with your left and look up. If this hurts your neck, look down at the ground instead.

4   Stay here for 5 breaths, inhaling to release a little and exhaling to twist deeper from your navel.

5   Press down into your feet to rise up to stand and step forward into Mountain Pose before switching your feet.

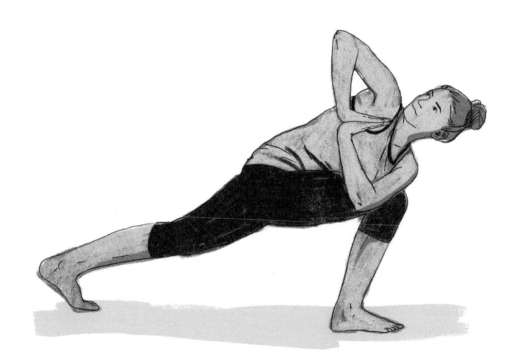

Revolved Extended Angle Pose

Parivrtta Parsvakonasana

Another cleansing twist, this pose revitalizes the internal organs, stokes the digestive fire, and improves digestion and elimination. Like all standing poses, it also strengthens and tones the legs.

QUALITY Grounding, energizing **EFFECT** Cleansing, heat, strength **PROPS** Block
GAZE To the ground for balance, or up to the sky

1 Begin in Mountain Pose (page 49) at the top of your mat. Inhale your arms up and exhale over your legs into a Standing Forward Bend (page 51). As you inhale, reach your left leg back behind you into a Low Lunge (page 53). Exhale as you bring your left knee to the ground, and inhale as you raise your arms up on either side of your head into a modified High Lunge (page 55).

2 Stack the joints by making sure your right knee is in line with your right ankle. This is important for stability. Place your left knee under your left hip.

3 Bring your hands together at your heart as if in prayer and begin to twist from the navel, hooking your left elbow to the outside of your right knee. Draw your right shoulder back to open your chest, and draw your thumbs to the center of your chest.

4 You can keep your left knee on the ground for balance, or tuck your toes under and lift your knee off the ground, drawing the right hip back. You can stay with your hands in prayer or open your arms wide with your left hand toward the ground and your right arm opening up toward the sky.

5 Take your gaze up and stay for 5 breaths. The inhale will be a bit constrained because of the twist, but you can release a bit to breathe in. Deepen the rotation with each exhale.

6 Release your hands down to frame your right foot and step your left foot up into a Standing Forward Bend. To switch sides, lunge back with the right leg.

7 When you've practiced on both sides, end in Mountain Pose.

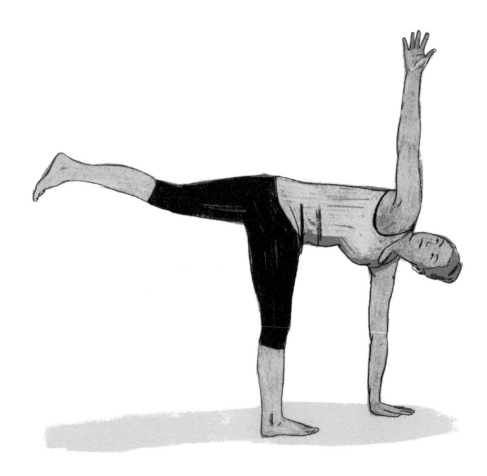

Revolved Half Moon Pose

Parivrtta Ardha Chandrasana

Head to the dark side of the moon. The revolved version of the beautiful Half Moon (page 81) is challenging and takes a while to feel comfortable in. (I'm still working on it after 25 years.) The benefits of mental and physical strength and stamina, open shoulders, and flexible hamstrings and spine, along with strong core muscles, outweigh the initial aversion you'll feel. Stay connected to the breath and find peace within the challenge. Make sure you have a block or two nearby.

QUALITY Grounding, energizing   EFFECT Strength, flexibility, cleansing, heat   PROPS Block
GAZE To the ground for balance or up to the extended hand

1   Begin in Mountain Pose (page 49) at the top of your mat. As you inhale, raise your arms above your head, and as you exhale, move into a Standing Forward Bend (page 51).

2   Shift your weight onto your right leg and reach your left leg straight up, parallel with the ground.

3   Place a block directly under your left hand in line with your left shoulder. Place your right hand on your right hip.

4   Begin to rotate your chest open to the right, twisting from your navel. Roll your shoulders back and down away from your ears to lengthen your neck and open your chest.

5   Reach down into your left hand, and open your right arm into the sky followed by your gaze.

6   Stay here for 3 to 5 breaths, breathing through the burn and relaxing the face and jaw.

7   Return to Standing Forward Bend with your left foot meeting the right and right hand meeting the left. Exhale through your mouth and move your hips from side to side before switching sides.

8   Finish by rising back up into Mountain Pose.

STANDING BALANCING POSES

Although simple looking, balancing poses are some of the most challenging. Standing on one leg calls our focus to one point, engaging and awakening new muscles, while we continue to breathe and stay calm. These poses build physical, emotional, and mental strength, balance, and confidence. They allow us to find our center and stay there throughout our day, no matter how busy we are or what challenges are placed in our path.

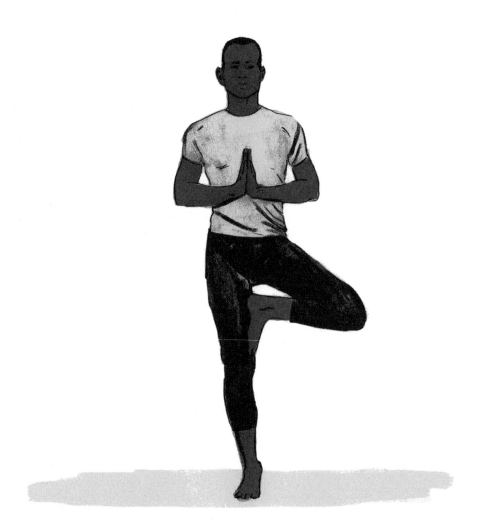

Tree Pose

Vrksasana

Tree Pose reconnects us to the earth and nature. With this pose, we draw up the nourishment and strength from the earth and generously offer ourselves back to the world. It makes us grounded and rooted.

QUALITY Grounding, **EFFECT** Balance, focus, stability, strength **PROPS** None **GAZE** Forward

1 Stand with your feet hip-distance apart, creating a stable base. On an exhale, soften your knees and release your tailbone down as you engage your thighs. Shift your weight onto your left foot and draw your right knee into your chest. (Feel free to stand at a wall and place your left hand there for support if you need it.)

2 Draw the sole of your right foot to the inside of your left inner thigh or calf, avoiding the knee joint. Roll your right knee open to the right from your hip joint. Place your hands together at your heart in prayer and balance for a breath or two, gazing at a still point in front of you.

3 Continue dropping your tailbone and engaging the left thigh. Lift up your lower belly for inner stability, and try reaching your arms up like branches reaching up into the sky.

4 Stay for 5 breaths before releasing your right foot and arms down into Mountain Pose (page 49), and switch sides.

VARIATION

For Extended Tree Pose, after finding your balance in Tree Pose, place your left hand on your left hip and reach for your big right toe with your right hand. Extend your right leg wide out to the right and extend your left arm out to the left along with your gaze for balance. Press through your left foot as you lift through the crown of your head. Hold for 3 to 5 breaths, and switch sides.

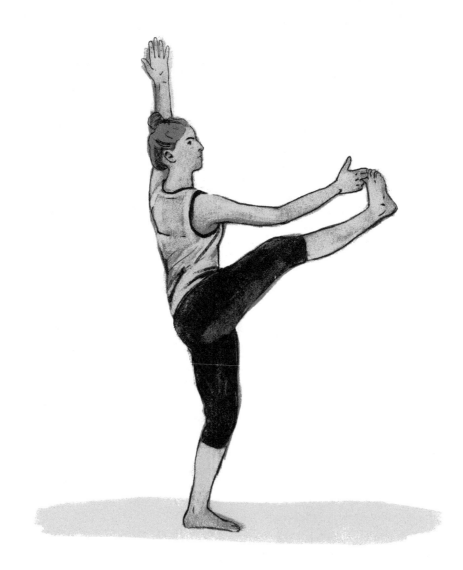

Standing One-Leg Balance Pose

Utthita Hasta Padangusthasana

This pose has all the stabilizing and strengthening attributes of Tree Pose (page 99), but is more mentally and physically challenging. It also provides a deep hamstring stretch. This is a pose to practice in preparation for more advanced arm balances and inversions.

QUALITY Balancing, grounding   **EFFECT** Flexibility, focus, strength   **PROPS** Strap   **GAZE** Forward

1   Begin in Mountain Pose (page 49) to establish a stable base. Shift your weight onto your left foot and hug your right knee into your chest. Roll your shoulders back and down your back and lift your chest. Find a still point of focus for your gaze out in front of you.

2   Place your left hand on your left hip and place your right arm in the inside of your right knee to reach for your big right toe with your middle and index fingers. Wrap your fingers and thumb around your toe.

3   Keeping your chest lifted and right shoulder back, begin to extend your right leg forward as far as it will go. Drop your right hip down, keeping it in line with the left hip.

4   Extend your left arm to the sky and stay here for 3 to 5 breaths, cultivating mental strength and stamina.

5   Return to Mountain Pose and switch sides.

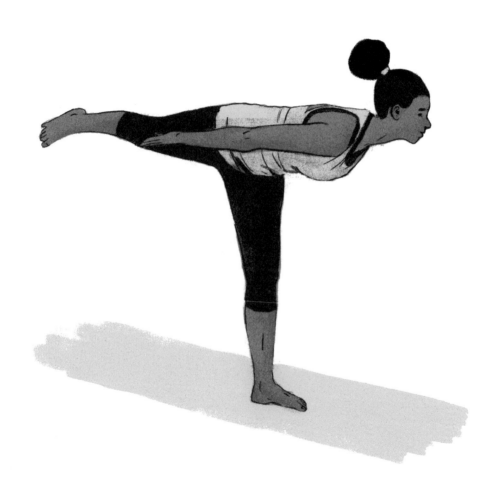

Warrior III Pose

Virabhadrasana III

This warrior pose cultivates balance as well as enhancing strength in the legs, buttocks, hips, abdominal muscles, and triceps. It also heightens mental focus and awakens the feeling of taking flight.

QUALITY Balancing, grounding   **EFFECT** Focus, energy, strength
PROPS Blocks   **GAZE** Forward and down

1   Begin in Mountain Pose (page 49) with your hands on your hips and your feet hip-distance apart. Shift your weight onto your right foot and tip your weight forward, extending your left leg straight back behind you so your whole torso and left leg are parallel with the ground. (If you feel a strain in your lower back, place your hands on blocks directly under your shoulders.)

2   Flex your left foot and lift your left thigh as you roll your left hip down so it is in line with your right.

3   Draw your navel in to support your spine, and lift your shoulders to open your chest as you reach back strongly with your arms. If this is too much, leave your hands on the blocks.

4   Draw your chin in slightly to lengthen your neck and gaze down and in front of you. Stay here for 3 to 5 breaths, feeling grounded and free.

5   Return to Mountain Pose and switch sides.

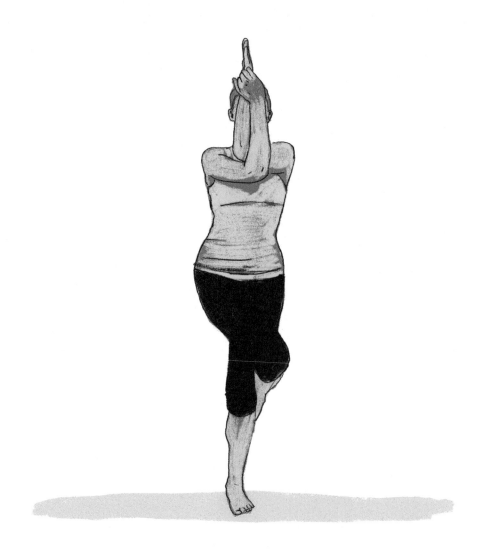

Eagle Pose

Garudasana

This balancing pose cultivates concentration and focus as well as the strength, poise, and lightness characteristic of the majestic bird of prey for which it is named. It opens the back body and tones the internal organs. Although the pose may initially feel uncomfortable, it's for stretching and strengthening the joints and bones.

QUALITY Balancing. Grounding   EFFECT Cleansing, focus, stability
PROPS None   GAZE Forward and down

1 Begin in Mountain Pose (page 49), and bend your knees deeply. Shift your weight onto your right foot. Lift your left leg up and wrap it around your right leg as if crossing your legs in a chair. See if you can hook your left foot behind your right ankle. If not, simply keep your legs crossed or place your left foot's toes on the ground outside the right foot for balance.

2 When you find your balance, hook your left elbow under your right elbow and weave your left forearm around your right one to join your palms.

3 Lift your elbows away from your knees with your spine long, and exhale to fold forward, hinging at the hips and reaching your elbows toward your knees.

4 Find a point of focus on the ground and stay for 3 to 5 breaths, cultivating consciousness and mindfulness by being completely present.

5 Unravel your arms and legs and return to Mountain Pose. Shake out your body a bit before switching legs.

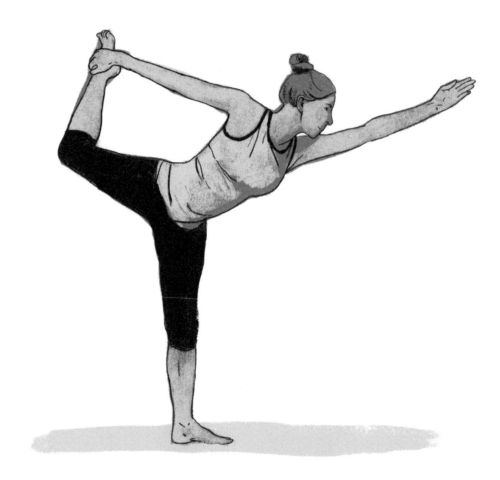

Dancer's Pose

Natarajasana

This exquisite pose cultivates the grace, beauty, strength, and flexibility of a dancer, stretching the body out in all directions at once! It symbolizes openness to the future while being rooted in the present and connected to the past. It stretches the front body— quadriceps, abdominals, chest, and shoulders—while strengthening the back body—buttocks, spine, and hamstrings.

QUALITY Grounding, energizing   EFFECT Flexibility, focus, grace, stability
PROPS Strap   GAZE Forward

1   Begin in Mountain Pose (page 49), with both feet firmly rooted on the ground. Shift your weight onto your right foot and bend your right knee, lifting your heel toward your left sit bone. Reach back with your left hand to grab the top of your right foot. Draw your heel closer to your seat, stretching your left quadriceps.

2   Place your right hand on your heart with your thumb and index finger touching, and find your breath before reaching forward with your right arm and back with your left foot.

3   Keep shifting your weight forward and up, maintaining balance by reaching your left leg back and up as you drop your left hip down in line with the right.

4   Stay for 3 to 5 five breaths, cultivating the courage to stay open.

5   Return to Mountain Pose before switching feet.

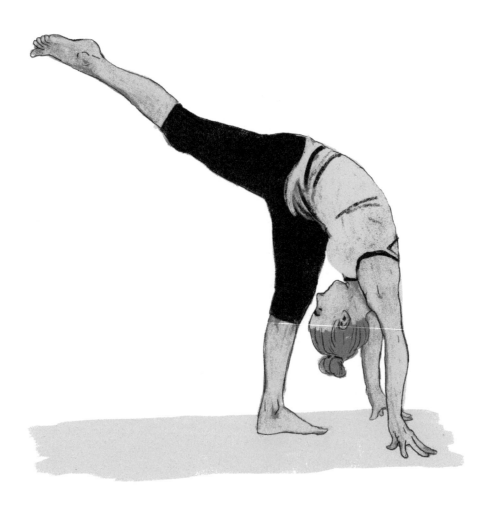

Standing Split Pose

Urdhva Prasarita Eka Padasana

Make sure you're fully warmed up through Sun Salutations (page 199) and some standing poses before practicing this all-around awesome asana. This challenging balancing pose stretches every muscle of your body. It's a great preparation for inversions such as Handstand.

QUALITY Grounding, calming, energizing **EFFECT** Balance, flexibility, strength
PROPS Blocks **GAZE** The ground

1 Begin in Mountain Pose (page 49), fully connected to your breath and body. As you inhale, lift your arms up above your head, and exhale while moving into Standing Forward Bend (page 51) with your hands on the ground or blocks.

2 Shift your weight onto your right foot, and lift your left leg straight up into the sky as far as it can go behind you. Release your head toward the ground and your face toward your right shin. Stay here for 5 breaths, going deeper into the pose with each breath.

3 Walk your hands as far back toward your right heel as you can, and energetically reach up with your left leg in the opposite direction.

4 Play with your balance by first taking your left hand to your right ankle and then your right hand to your right ankle. As you do this, lift your gaze and chest a bit and look forward at the ground.

5 When you are ready, release your left leg and return to Mountain Pose, before switching legs.

CORE WORK AND ARM BALANCES

Although yoga's impressive arm balances look like they require a lot of arm strength, they're actually possible through a strong core and inner strength and confidence. These take time and require risk-taking and patience. Once mastered, these are the poses that will make inversions accessible and fun.

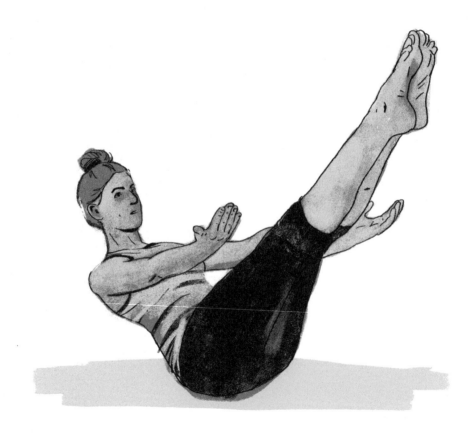

Boat Pose

Navasana

Practicing this pose is like having a cup of coffee! It wakes you up from the inside out to jump-start your day and make you feel like anything is possible. The challenge is to stay with the pose as you burn. The best pose for strengthening the core muscles, it also stretches and lengthens the back body. Yogis practice this pose to stimulate digestion and elimination, and to relieve stress.

QUALITY Energizing **EFFECT** Cleansing, heat, strength **PROPS** None **GAZE** Forward

1 Begin in a seated position on your mat. Hug your knees into your chest with your hands under your knees, balancing on your sit bones.

2 Lift your shins parallel with the ground, and lean back a bit with your hands supporting the backs of your knees. Lift your chest up and shoulders back into a supported Boat Pose.

3 Shift your weight slightly forward to the fronts of your sit bones, and straighten your legs as far as they'll extend. Let go of your legs, and reach your arms forward in line with your knees.

4 Look forward and stay here for 5 breaths, feeling your aliveness! You'll experience some shaking, which is totally normal. Use your abdominal muscles to stay lifted rather than your back muscles, shoulders, or neck, and release your jaw.

5 Lower onto your back and hug your knees into your chest before rocking back up to sit.

VARIATION

In step 4, if you feel ready to challenge yourself after 3 breaths, exhale and lower down 2 to 3 inches from the ground into Half Boat. Tuck your chin in toward your chest, and stretch your legs long out in front of you with your toes pointed, drawing your navel in. Hold your exhale, and then inhale to rise back up into Boat Pose with your knees slightly bent. Repeat 3 to 5 times, exhaling to lower down and inhaling to rise up. When you're done, lower down onto your back and hug your knees into your chest before rocking back up to sit.

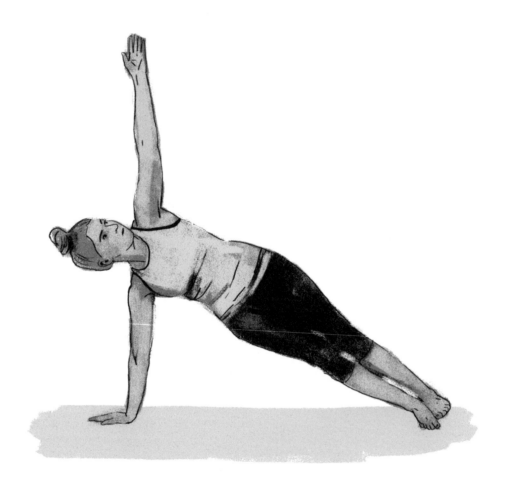

Side Plank Pose

Vasisthasana

A powerful arm balance on its own, Side Plank and its variations are great way to prepare for more advanced arm balances. Side Planks mimic the standing poses, but are done on the side, therefore challenging your perspective, mental focus, and balance. They strengthen the arms, wrists, shoulders, abdominal muscles, and spine. The variations include hip openers, back bends, and hamstring stretches.

QUALITY Energizing, grounding   **EFFECT** Stability, strength   **PROPS** None   **GAZE** Up

1 Begin in Downward-Facing Dog (page 37) and move into a Plank Pose (page 39), reaching back though your heels and forward with your chest. Lift your ribs and navel. Shift your right hand to the center of your mat and roll over onto the outer edge of your right foot. Stack your left foot directly on top of your right, flexing strongly through both your feet.

2 Lift your hips so they're in line with your shoulders. When you feel stable, lift your left arm straight up to the sky.

3 Stay for up to 5 breaths, twisting your right hip slightly up toward the sky and drawing your bottom ribs in. Gaze either at the wall in front of you or up toward your left hand.

4 With all variations, return to Plank Pose and rest in Child's Pose (page 35), before repeating on the left side.

VARIATION

If this pose puts too much pressure on your right wrist, lower your right shin to the ground with your right knee directly under your right hip for a Supported Side Plank.

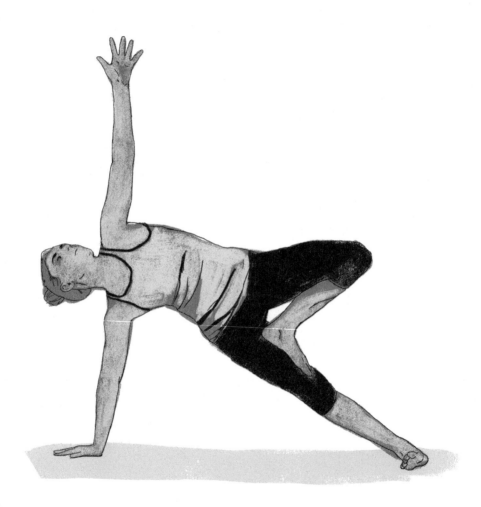

Side Plank with Tree Pose

For a challenge, explore this variation of Side Plank (page 115). Side Plank with Tree offers the balancing qualities of Tree Pose (page 99) with the upper-body strength enhancement of Side Plank and takes both poses to the next level. It's a great hip opener and a great prep for more advanced arm balances.

QUALITY Energizing, grounding   **EFFECT** Flexibility, stability, strength   **PROPS** None   **GAZE** Up

Begin in Side Plank first and find your stability. Bend your left knee and open your hip to the left, placing the sole of your left foot on your inner right thigh. Press your right thigh into your left foot and lift your hips to avoid sinking or putting too much pressure in your right wrist.

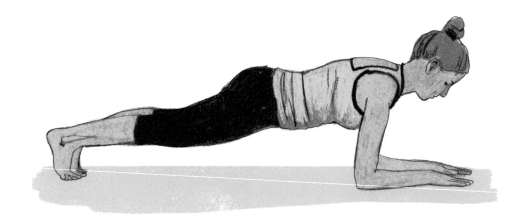

Forearm Plank Pose

Phalakasana

A favorite in many workouts and a staple in yoga, this pose is great preparation for inversions such as Forearm Stand (page 131) and Headstand (page 135). It cultivates strength in your arms and core so you can support the head and whole body, upside down!

QUALITY Energizing, grounding   EFFECT Strength, focus, heat
PROPS None   GAZE Forward and down

1   Begin on your hands and knees. Lower your forearms so they rest on the ground, with your elbows directly under your shoulders and your wrists aligned with your elbows. Spread your hands wide and press down into your thumbs and index fingers as you roll your shoulders away from your ears.

2   Stretch your right leg back, lifting your right knee off the ground and flexing your foot. Strongly lift up through your navel and lengthen the left leg back to join the right.

3   Reach forward with your chest and soften the back of your heart down as you lift your ribs and front body.

4   Draw your chin in slightly to lengthen the back of your neck, but look slightly forward. Stay here for 5 breaths. Feel the strength and steadiness of your body affecting the strength of your mind.

5   Bend your knees and send your hips back to your heels into Child's Pose (page 35).

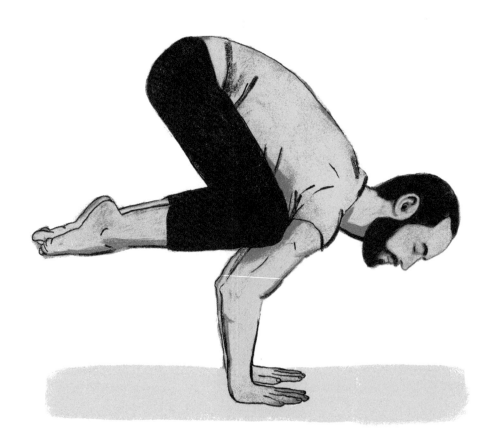

Crow Pose

Bakasana

Most arm balances are named after creatures of flight. As the name suggests, this pose awakens our ability to fly. It's the foundation for all other arm balances. When we engage and lift our navel up, our inner wings soar and we can let go. This pose will help you overcome fear and develop confidence. It tones the internal organs and strengthens the arms and core muscles while improving focus, balance, and concentration. Using a block for support is a great way to start.

QUALITY Energizing, grounding   **EFFECT** Focus, strength   **PROPS** Block   **GAZE** Forward and down

1 Begin in Garland Pose (page 85) with your feet close together, your elbows inside your knees, and your hands at your heart as if in prayer.

2 Place your hands on the ground a few inches in front of you and reach your torso forward so your knees come high up to your upper arms.

3 Shift your weight forward onto the balls of your feet so your elbows are in line with your wrists. Grip your fingers into your mat to protect your wrists.

4 Hug your knees into your upper arms and lift your right foot off the ground with your heel toward your sit bone. Focus your gaze on the ground and a few inches forward. As you inhale, draw your tailbone down and in, lifting up through your navel, and then exhale the left foot up to join the right.

5 Practice holding for 3 to 5 breaths. Release back to a Garland Pose or Child's Pose (page 35) before trying again.

VARIATION

If Crow Pose is too challenging, place a block toward the top of your mat. Come to perch on your tiptoes on the wide side of the block, and follow the steps above but keep your toes together and your knees wide. Place your hands on the ground and you'll have some extra lift in your hips to easily shift your weight forward and play with balance. Follow the rest of the steps above.

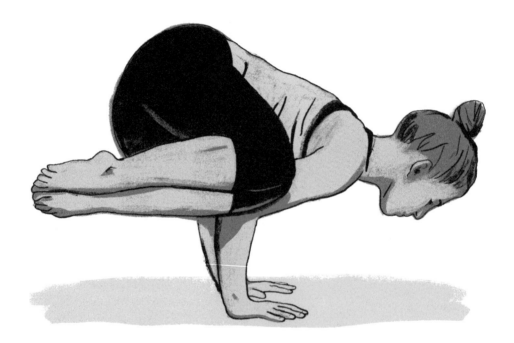

Side Crow Pose

Parsva Bakasana

Side Crow is the rotated version of Crow (page 121). It's a more challenging version that amplifies all its benefits with a cleansing twist and added mental and physical challenges. It can also be practiced with a block under your feet for extra lift.

QUALITY Energizing, grounding   EFFECT Cleansing, heat, stability, strength
PROPS Block   GAZE Forward and down

1 Begin in Mountain Pose (page 49) with your feet together, approaching this challenge with confidence. Inhale while you raise your arms above your head and dive forward over your legs into a Standing Forward Bend (page 51).

2 Bend your knees deeply, keeping your knees and ankles together, and lift your heels up so you are perching on the balls of your feet. Balance on your tiptoes, with your heels touching your buttocks and your hands at your heart as if in prayer.

3 Keep your shins facing forward, but twist your torso to the right as much as possible, and place your hands on the ground with your left elbow on the outside of your right thigh.

4 Press both hands firmly into the ground, and roll your right shoulder back in line with the left. Bend your elbows, making a shelf to place your legs on. Shift your weight forward, keeping your inner thighs together, and lift your feet off the ground as you focus your gaze forward.

5 Stay here for 3 to 5 breaths, and release into a Standing Forward Bend.

6 Repeat on the left side, and then return to Mountain Pose.

INVERSIONS AND PREPS

Although they can seem scary at first, inversions include some of the most powerful poses in yoga. Known as the fountain of youth, they're believed to reverse the aging process by flooding the brain with nutrients and clearing out stagnation. They're energizing as well as calming, and seen as an antidote to depression in therapeutic yoga. Make sure you're fully warmed up and have practiced plenty of standing poses before trying to go upside down.

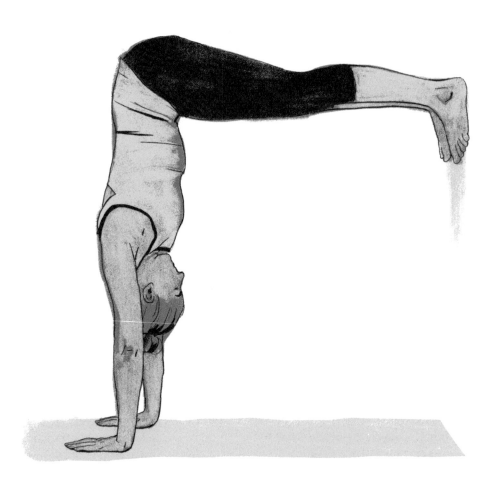

L-Shaped Handstand Pose

Adho Mukha Vrksasana

Handstands can be exhilarating, and are meant to be a practice. The goal is to take the first step and gradually build the upper-body strength and inner lift needed to stay upside down. The L-Shaped Handstand, practiced at a wall, is a great way to start your inversion practice.

QUALITY Energizing, grounding **EFFECT** Flexibility, stability, strength
PROPS None **GAZE** Toward the wall and slightly up

1 Place the front of your mat against the wall. Come onto your hands and knees, with your toes tucked under and the soles of your feet pressing into the wall. Lift your knees but keep them bent, with your chest pressing toward the tops of your thighs into a modified Downward-Facing Dog (page 37).

2 Lift your right foot and place it up the wall in line with your hips. Press your right foot strongly into the wall and hands into the ground, with your shoulders over your wrists. Lift your left foot to the same height as your right foot, and straighten your knees so your legs make an L-shape. Draw your chin into your chest and your front ribs into your back to support your lower back and lengthen your spine.

3 Look up toward your feet and lift your right leg straight up with your toes flexed. Switch your feet, placing the right foot to meet the left and lifting the left leg straight up. Place it back down and walk or jump both feet down to the mat. Rest in Child's Pose (page 35) before trying again.

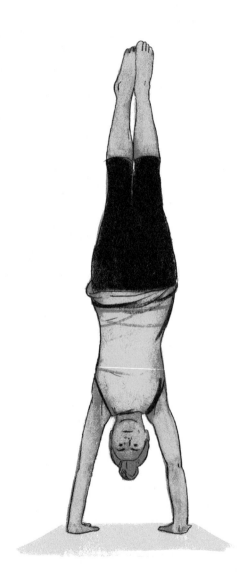

Handstand Pose

Adho Mukha Vrksasana

When you feel ready, explore hopping up into Handstand. In Sanskrit, "handstand" translates to "upside-down tree," so you're bound to feel a bit uprooted. Spiritually, this pose is used to break free from limited thinking and habitual patterns. Try practicing it whenever you feel stuck.

QUALITY Energizing **EFFECT** Cleansing, focus, strength, tranquility **PROPS** None **GAZE** Down

1 Place the front of your mat near a wall. Come onto your hands and knees with your hands about 6 inches away from the wall. Spread your hands wide and grip your mat with your fingertips as you roll your shoulders down and away from your ears. Tuck your toes under and exhale as you go into Downward-Facing Dog (page 37).

2 Look forward between your hands and walk your feet forward so your shoulders are over your wrists and hips over your shoulders.

3 Inhale while you move your right leg up so it's parallel with the ground with your right hip pointing down. Bend your left knee and come onto the ball of your left foot.

4 Using your exhale, strongly press off the ball of your left foot and hop your heel toward your buttocks to send your right leg up the wall. Do this a few times until your right heel is on the wall and you can lengthen your left leg up to meet your right.

5 Once you're upside down, stay for 3 to 5 breaths. Focus your gaze on the ground between your hands or draw your chin toward your chest, and rest your head between your upper arms and look out in front of you.

6 Flex your feet to engage your thighs, and roll them in as your draw your front ribs in to support your lower back.

7 When you're ready to come down, rest in Child's Pose (page 35) for a few breaths. Slowly rise up to sit with your head coming up last to avoid getting light-headed.

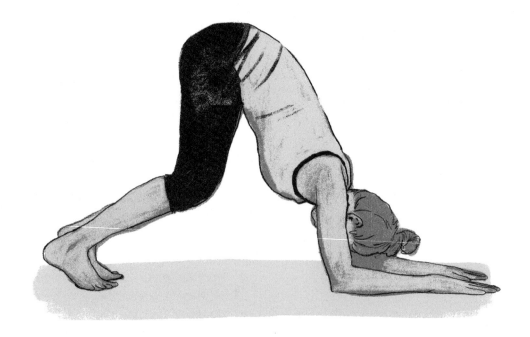

Dolphin Pose

Ardha Pincha Mayurasana

Dolphin Pose is a great preparation for Forearm Stand (page 131) and Headstand (page 135). It helps develop strength and flexibility in the arms, shoulders, and chest to support your head and the delicate vertebrae of the neck. It's also a good way to prepare for backbends, opening the back of the heart, shoulders, thoracic spine, and legs.

QUALITY Grounding, calming   EFFECT Strength, flexibility, stability
PROPS None   GAZE Toward your feet

1 Begin on your hands and knees. Move your forearms down to the ground, with your elbows under your shoulders and your wrists in line with your elbows. Roll down your inner wrists and press your thumbs down as you rotate your shoulders back and away from your ears to widen your chest and collarbone.

2 Tuck your toes under and lift your knees off the ground and your hips toward the sky.

3 Keep your knees slightly bent and press your chest toward your thighs as you continue to draw your shoulders away from your ears. Draw your chin in toward your throat to lengthen the back of your neck, and stay here for up to 5 breaths.

4 Eventually lengthen your legs by straightening your knees, keeping your chest and shoulders open. Play with lifting one leg up and then the other, before releasing down into Child's Pose (page 35).

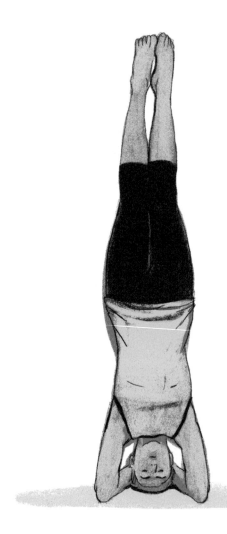

Forearm Stand Pose

Pincha Mayurasana

In Sanskrit, this pose translates to "Peacock's Tail," symbolizing the exquisite nature of this position. Along with strengthening the upper body, this pose opens the heart and lungs, focuses the mind, and deepens concentration. A peacock's tail appears to be decorated with many eyes, so it's no coincidence that you'll feel more awake when in this gorgeous shape. While practicing, visualize someone you love, since this pose stirs up devotion and is meant to be an offering.

QUALITY Energizing **EFFECT** Chest-opening, focus, strength, tranquility
PROPS Block **GAZE** Forward and down

1 Bring the front of your mat to a wall, place your fingers a few inches back from the wall, and follow the steps for Dolphin Pose (page 129). When you're ready to fly up, lift your gaze between your hands and walk your feet forward on your tiptoes. Be sure to keep your hips in line with your shoulders.

2 Lift your right leg up. Bend your left knee as you inhale, and use your exhale to hop your left leg off the ground to meet your right leg up on the wall. This may take a few attempts. The key is to lift your left leg and draw your left heel toward your left sit bone to build momentum to get your right leg to the wall. Once you get your right leg up, bring your left leg up to meet your right.

3 Stay here for up to 5 breaths, keeping your heels on the wall. Flex your feet, rolling your inner thighs in to widen and lengthen your lower back. Keep your gaze forward and between your hands, and draw your shoulders back to open your chest. If you want to play with balance, draw your bottom ribs in and navel back, and lift one foot and then the other off the wall.

4 When you're ready to come down, lead with your left leg and come down gracefully into Child's Pose (page 35).

5 Repeat with the left side to cultivate equilibrium in the legs.

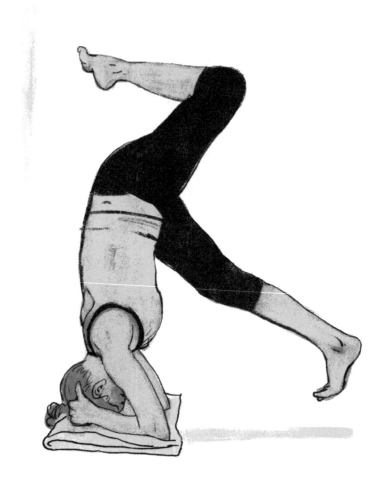

Headstand Prep Pose

Ardha Sirsasana

Known as the king of the asanas, Headstand is a master pose that awakens the crown chakra, or energy center, leading to enlightenment. Ancient yogis used Headstand to stimulate the pineal gland, which they believed would release powerful antiaging and antidepressant chemicals. To prepare for this asana, you need a solid foundation in the arms and sufficient strength to support all the weight of your body on your head. Practicing this Headstand Prep is an important first step.

QUALITY Grounding, energizing   **EFFECT** Cleansing, focus, strength, tranquility
PROPS Blanket   **GAZE** Forward

1 Come onto your hands and knees, facing the wall and about 2 inches from the wall. Place your forearms on the ground with your elbows under your shoulders, and interlace your fingers with your pinky fingers tucked in, creating a "crown" for your head. Roll your shoulders back and away from your ears and make sure your shoulders are in line with your elbows. Place the crown of your head on the ground and wrap your hands around the back of your head with your thumbs at the base of your skull.

2 Tuck your toes under and lift your knees off the ground, lifting your hips up toward the sky. Draw your chin in toward your chest but keep your head off the ground.

3 Walk your feet as far forward as they will go so your hips are in line and above your shoulders. Practice lifting one foot and then the other by bending at the knee and reaching your heel close toward your buttocks and toward the wall, engaging your core muscles to stay lifted.

4 Stay in this pose for up to 5 breaths.

5 Release into Child's Pose (page 35).

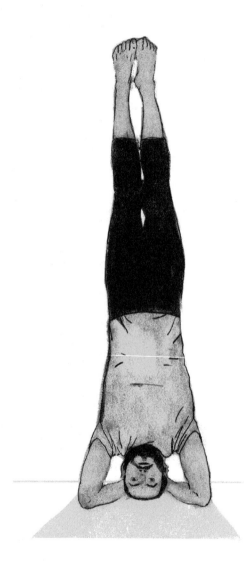

Headstand Pose

Sirsasana

When you're ready to attempt Headstand, start by bringing your mat to a wall. You can fold the edge of your mat to create extra padding for your head. Make sure you're fully warmed up, especially in your core, hamstrings, and shoulders. It's important not to kick up into this pose, so cultivate a lot of inner strength and ease into it. Be careful not to strain your neck. Avoid this pose if you have any neck injuries.

QUALITY Grounding, energizing   EFFECT Cleansing, focus, strength, tranquility
PROPS None   GAZE Forward

1   Come onto your hands and knees facing the wall and about 2 inches from the wall. Place your forearms on the ground with your elbows under your shoulders, and interlace your fingers with your pinky fingers tucked in. Roll your shoulders back and away from your ears and make sure they're in line with your elbows. Place the crown of your head on the ground and wrap your hands around the back of your head with your thumbs at the base of your skull.

2   Press your forearms deeply into the ground as you tuck your toes under and lift your knees off the ground. Shift most of your weight into your forearms rather than your head.

3   Draw your shoulders away from your ears and your shoulder blades in as your walk your feet forward until you're in a V-shape on your head.

4   Bend your knees and draw them into your chest. Lift your feet off the ground one at a time. Slowly lengthen your legs up the wall and hold for up to 5 breaths.

5   Flex your feet to activate your legs, and roll your inner thighs inward. Continue to reach your legs up as you root down into your forearms with only about 25 percent of your weight on your head to begin.

6   When you're ready to come down, slowly bend your knees with your feet on the wall, and draw your knees into your chest before releasing into Child's Pose (page 35).

7   Come up to sit on your heels for a few breaths before trying again.

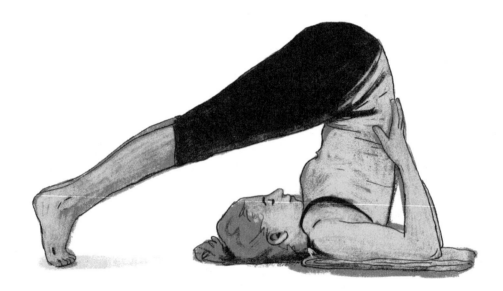

Plow Pose

Halasana

While Headstand may be the king, Shoulder Stand is the queen and mother of the asanas! Plow Pose is prep for Shoulder Stand (page 139), so work this pose until you feel comfortable moving on to a full Shoulder Stand. The neck and the cervical vertebrae are vulnerable here, so place a blanket under your shoulders to relieve pressure on the neck. This pose stretches the spine and whole back body, or back of the body.

QUALITY Calming, energizing   **EFFECT** Balance, cleansing, tranquility   **PROPS** Blanket   **GAZE** Inward

1 Start by taking a firm blanket and folding it in thirds and thirds again to form a rectangle that's the width of your mat, about 3 to 4 feet long and 3 to 4 inches thick. Lay it on your mat a few feet away from the end. Fold the mat over the blanket and lie down with your head on the ground and your shoulders at the edge of the padding. This way, there should be some space between your neck and the ground.

2 Bend your knees and lengthen your arms by your sides with your hands pressing into the ground by your hips.

3 Using your abdominal muscles, draw your knees into your chest and lift your hips off the ground as you roll onto your shoulders. Lengthen your legs over your head with your thighs vertical to the ground.

4 Interlace your fingers together and roll your upper arms and shoulders out and down. Drawing your chin to your chest, press your arms into the ground as you flex your feet behind you and press your thighs up into the backs of your legs.

5 Stay here for up to 5 breaths with your gaze toward your navel. Release down onto your back or move on to Shoulder Stand.

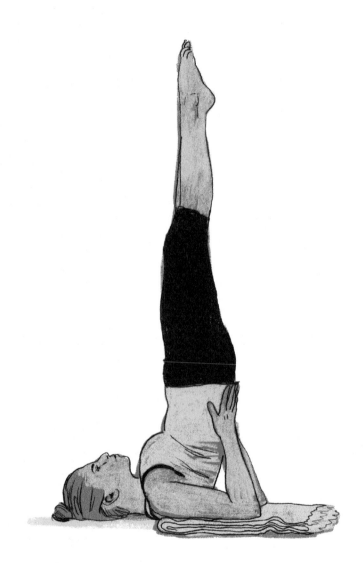

Shoulder Stand Pose

Salamba Sarvangasana

Practicing Shoulder Stand every day is meant to lead to increased physical, mental, and emotional health and well-being. In Sanskrit, it translates to "Supported All Parts." It nourishes and purifies every part and system of the body, regulates emotions, and calms the mind. By contracting the throat, this pose is thought to stimulate the thyroid and parathyroid glands, which are responsible for metabolism and growth. Given the supported position, this inversion can be practiced for longer than most. Practice this asana before your final relaxation or whenever you need a mini reboot.

QUALITY Calming **EFFECT** Cleansing, tranquility **PROPS** Blanket **GAZE** Inward

1   Follow all the steps for Plow Pose (page 137). Once comfortable there, release your hands and bend your elbows to place your hands on your lower back. Using your abdominal muscles, bend your knees and shift your weight into your elbows and hands, with your hips in line with your shoulders and your heels near your buttocks.

2   Slowly unfurl your body up into a vertical line. Straighten your legs with your feet reaching up toward the sky and your elbows pressing deeply into the ground, keeping the weight off your neck.

3   Stay here for 10 to 25 breaths, keeping your gaze toward your navel. If you feel too much strain in your neck, send your hips back toward your hands and lower your legs halfway.

4   When you're ready to come down, lower back down into Plow Pose. Bend your knees around your ears for a breath or two before anchoring your hands by your sides. Slowly release down, vertebra by vertebra.

5   Arrive on your back with bent knees and your feet on the ground. Stay here for a moment before rolling over to your right side and slowly rising up to sit.

BACKBENDS

B.K.S Iyengar, a great yoga master, says that backbends address fear. One reason for this is that they open and expose all the vulnerable parts of our bodies, including our hearts. By opening the heart chakra, a spiritual energy center along the spine, backbends also awaken qualities such as compassion, love, and joy. Take plenty of time to warm up through Sun Salutations (page 199) before practicing these heart-opening poses.

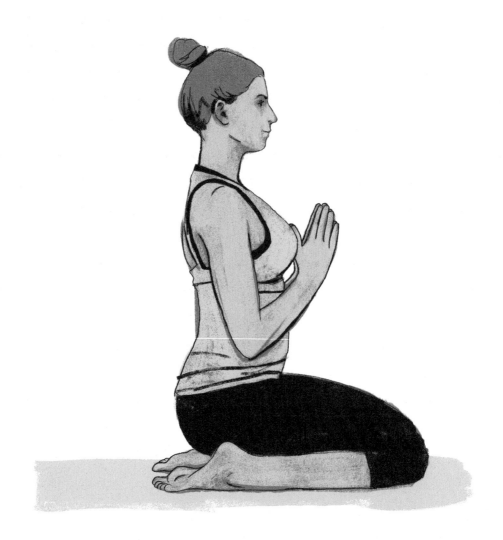

Hero's Pose

Virasana

Although not technically a backbend, this pose is an important preparation and meditation posture. It stretches the quadriceps, knees, ankles, groins, and psoas major muscle along the spine, and lengthens the spine, all of which are important for a backbend practice. As the name also suggests, the pose cultivates the bravery needed to stay open to all of life.

QUALITY Grounding   EFFECT Flexibility, stability, tranquility   PROPS Block or blanket
GAZE Forward and down

1 Begin on your shins, sitting on your heels. Place a blanket under your shins if needed.

2 Lean forward with your hands on the ground. Widen your feet about hip-distance apart and roll your heels open to the outside edges of your feet, keeping your knees together. Use your hands to draw your calf muscles out to the sides. Slowly lift your hips back and sit between your heels. If you feel any pressure in your knees, place a block between your heels, wide-side up, and sit on the block.

3 Distribute your weight equally between your sit bones and sit up tall. Draw your shoulders back and wrap your shoulder blades around your upper spine to broaden your chest and heart. Draw in the bottom ribs to lift out of your lower back and feel the back of the heart lift as well.

4 Slide your hands to the top of your thighs and breathe. Tip your chin toward your chest to lengthen the back of your neck. Drop your gaze toward the tip of your nose and stay for 5 to 10 breaths or longer.

5 You can also do a breathing practice or meditation (see chapters 5 and 6) while in this pose. When you're ready to come out of the position, come onto your hands and knees. Stretch one leg back and then the other to return the blood flow to your legs before moving on to your next pose.

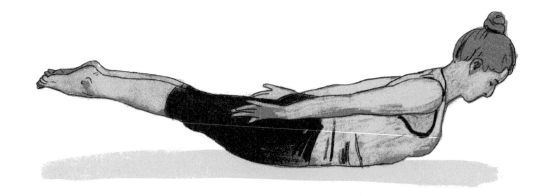

Locust Pose

Shalabhasana

This is a powerful pose for correcting poor, slouching posture by lifting the shoulders, stretching the chest, and strengthening the whole back body and spine. This pretty pose is also believed to stimulate digestion, elimination, and fertility. Practicing it regularly will help prepare you for some of the deeper backbends.

QUALITY Energizing, grounding **EFFECT** Strength, stimulation, open chest
PROPS Blanket **GAZE** Forward and up

1 Begin by lying facedown on your mat. Place a blanket under your hip bones if they're sensitive. Place your arms down on the ground by your sides and your forehead to the ground with your chin tucked in toward your chest.

2 Press down with the tops of your feet and hamstrings and stretch your arms back toward your feet, and begin to lift your head, shoulders, chest, and upper ribs off the ground. Keep your chin tucked slightly in to protect your neck.

3 Lift your legs off the ground using your inner thighs, and stretch your body up by pressing your pelvis and belly down.

4 Stay here for 3 to 5 breaths, with your gaze on the ground a few inches in front of you. Draw your legs into each other and widen your chest by drawing your shoulder blades back and closer together. When you're ready, lower down to the mat with your cheek to one side.

VARIATIONS

1 Begin the same way, but interlace your hands behind your back to stretch wide across your chest. Bring your shoulder blades together and draw your hands toward your feet.

2 Begin and end the same way, but extend your arms forward while in the pose to stretch the sides of the body and strengthen your upper back.

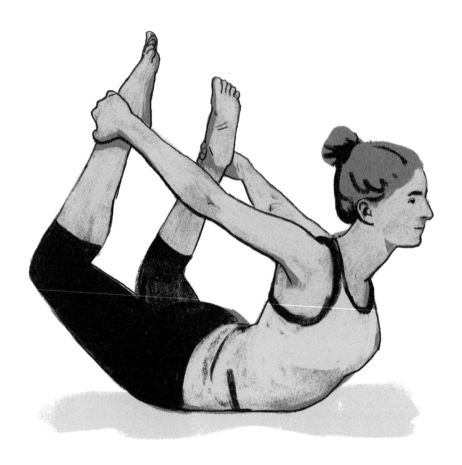

Bow Pose

Dhanurasana

Similar to Locust Pose (page 145), Bow Pose is a bit more advanced, requiring openness in the front of the body to reach all the way back for your ankles. An intense backbend, this pose feels like drawing back an arrow into a bow before shooting, and calls for a lot of mental focus and effort. Like all backbends, it strengthens the entire back body while stretching the whole front body. It's also thought to relieve menstrual discomfort and respiratory difficulties. Plus, it improves your mood!

QUALITY Energizing   **EFFECT** Flexibility, stability, strength,   **PROPS** Blanket   **GAZE** Forward and up

1 Begin by lying facedown on your mat, placing a blanket under your hip bones if they're sensitive. Place your arms down by your sides and your forehead down on the ground with your chin toward your chest. Draw your pubic bone up to your navel and your tailbone down toward your feet to lengthen and protect your lower back.

2 Bend your knees, bringing your heels up and back toward your buttocks. Reach back with your hands for your ankles, rolling your upper arms out and keeping your knees hip-distance apart.

3 Flex your feet and press your ankles into your hands, using your legs to lift your chest off the ground.

4 Shift your weight onto your belly and lift your thighs, lifting your legs and chest higher up as you press down into your belly and draw your tailbone down.

5 The breath will be a bit labored, but do your best to not hold your breath here. Stay for 5 breaths, inhaling to rise a little more and exhaling to release for 5 breaths. Rest before rising up one or two more times.

6 Come out of the pose by sliding your hands back alongside your rib cage and pressing your hips toward your heels into Child's Pose (page 35).

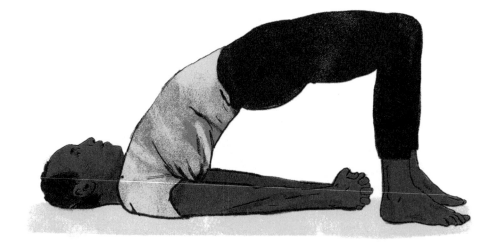

Half Wheel Pose

Setu Bandhasana

Full Wheel (page 151) is the apex of backbends, opening the heart wide open and stimulating full expression of the self. Although it is an advanced pose, kids seem to drop into it effortlessly with their flexible bodies and minds! You want to gradually work up to this pose with patience and persistence by practicing Half Wheel first. This will help you avoid injury to your lower back, wrists, shoulders, and neck. Half Wheel also opens up the chest, shoulders, hip flexors, and thighs, strengthening the back.

QUALITY Grounding **EFFECT** Flexibility, strength, tranquility **PROPS** Block **GAZE** Inward

1 Lie down on your back and bend your knees with your feet hip-distance apart and your heels close to your buttocks. Place your arms by your sides. Widen your heels and turn your toes in slightly. This widens the sacrum and narrows the hip points to protect your lower back from injury.

2 Root down into the mounds of your big toes. Inhale to lift your hips and chest up toward the sky, keeping your feet anchored and your knees pressing toward each other. Scoot your shoulders under you to widen your chest and interlace your fingers, drawing your palms together under your spine. Press down into the ground with your arms and feet to lift up your pelvis and chest.

3 Allow your gaze to focus on your heart center. Deepen your breathing into your chest, expanding your rib cage for 5 breaths.

4 When you're ready to come down, release your hips to the ground and drop your knees toward each other to ease the lower back. You can slowly swing your knees from side to side to gently massage your spine.

5 Repeat once or twice before moving on to a Full Wheel.

VARIATION

If this pose feels too intense on the lower back, place a block under your sacrum with your arms by your sides in a Supported Bridge, a more restorative version of Half Wheel.

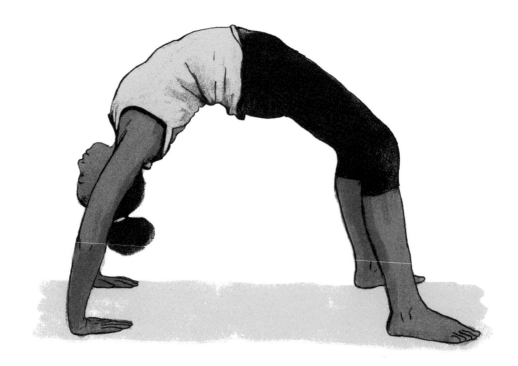

Full Wheel Pose

Urdhva Dhanurasana

This is the most joyful of poses, releasing held energy as it blows open the lungs and heart! It's great to practice during the darker months of winter, because it relieves the blues and lifts the spirit. This pose keeps the ego in check, requiring you to be aware of and honor your limitations while maintaining proper alignment.

QUALITY Energizing   **EFFECT** Flexibility, heat, lifted spirit, strength   **PROPS** None   **GAZE** Forward

1   Lie down on your back and bend your knees with your feet hip-distance apart and your heels close to your buttocks. Place your arms by your sides. Widen your heels and draw your toes in slightly. This widens the sacrum and narrows the hip points to protect your lower back from injury.

2   Reach your arms straight up and bend your elbows to plant the palms of your hands on the ground on either side of your head. Place your fingers under the tips of your shoulders and point your elbows straight up.

3   Exhale to root down into your feet and hands, and rise up to the crown of your head, drawing your elbows in and keeping them in line with your shoulders. Breathe in and draw your knees directly over your ankles. Exhale to press down equally into your hands and feet to straighten your arms and legs.

4   Keep drawing your knees and elbows in, and feel free to walk your feet toward your hands until you feel equal weight on your hands and feet.

5   Drop your gaze back to the ground between your hands, and stay here for up to 5 breaths. Release down by first drawing your chin into your chest to lengthen the back of your neck, and then slowly placing the back of your head on the ground, followed by your upper back, middle back, and lower back.

6   Place one hand on your belly and the other on your heart, and feel the energy pulsing through your body. Avoid drawing your knees straight into your chest as a counter pose because it's too extreme, especially if you plan on repeating the pose.

7   Repeat one or two more times, before slowly swinging your knees from side to side to neutralize and massage your spine.

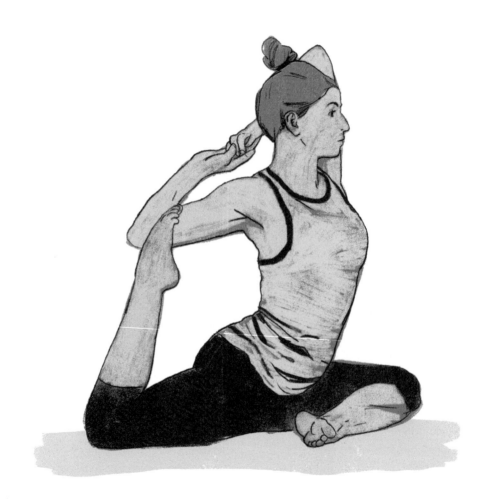

King Pigeon Pose

Eka Pada Rajakapotasana

This big, beautiful backbend pose symbolizes royalty. Make sure you're fully warmed up with backbends and open standing poses before you begin.

QUALITY Energizing, grounding **EFFECT** Flexibility, stability, tranquility
PROPS Blanket, strap **GAZE** Forward and up

1 Begin in Downward-Facing Dog (page 37). Reach your right leg up and bend your right knee to roll open your hip as you draw your right shoulder down. Keeping your knee bent, exhale to swing your right shin forward so it's parallel with the front edge of your mat. Flex your foot to protect your knee, and open your hip by drawing your knee a bit wider than your right hip. If your right hip lifts off the ground, place a rolled-up blanket or block under your hip.

2 Walk your hands back to either side of your hips. Roll your right hip back and left hip forward to create symmetry in the pelvis.

3 Tuck your left toes under and reach back with your left heel, grounding your pelvis down to lengthen your spine. Draw your shoulders back to open your chest and arch your back. Gently draw your chin into your chest to lengthen the back of your neck, and focus your gaze forward and slightly up. You're now in Seated Pigeon (page 207).

4 Bend your left knee and reach for the top of your left foot with your left hand, drawing your heel down toward your hip. To balance, draw your ribs and navel in, and lift your right arm up to the sky. Draw your left shoulder and hip forward and right shoulder back.

5 Lift your right arm and bend your right elbow with your hand reaching back toward your shoulder blades. Bend your left knee and reach back for the top of your left foot with your left hand. Slip the left foot into the space of your left inner elbow, and grab your right hand with your left arch back.

6 Stay here for 5 to 8 breaths and release down into Resting Pigeon (page 207), with your arms stretched forward or folded under your forehead for 3 breaths.

7 Step back into Downward-Facing Dog, and repeat with the left leg.

SUPINE TWISTS AND STRETCHES

Supine poses calm the mind and relieve stress and anxiety along with strain and stiffness from the body. They're a wonderful way to receive some of yoga's greatest benefits. You can practice these as a yoga beginner, while recovering from illness or injury, or after any type of strenuous workout.

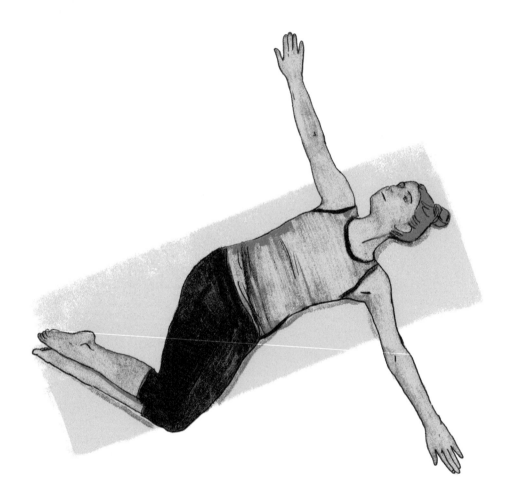

Supine Twist Pose

Supta Ardha Matsyendrasana

This simple reclined twist relieves tension in the lower back, sciatica, and shoulder and neck strain. Like other twists, it increases energy and is thought to stimulate digestion and elimination and calm the mind and nervous system.

QUALITY Calming **EFFECT** Flexibility, relaxation, tranquility
PROPS None **GAZE** Toward extended hand

1 Begin by lying on your back and hugging your knees to your chest. Take a few breaths here to allow your body to sink into the ground, releasing your lower back.

2 Keeping your knees together, press the outside of your right knee with your left hand to push both knees toward the ground on your left side, twisting as you exhale. Inhale to open your right arm wide out to the side in line with your right shoulder. Release your right ear toward the ground and gaze out past your right hand.

3 If your knees do not easily come to the ground, place a folded blanket or block under your left knee. Try to keep both shoulders on the ground.

4 Stay here for 8 to 10 breaths, twisting and releasing deeper with each exhale.

5 Bring your knees back up together and hug them to your chest for a couple of breaths, before releasing your knees to the right and twisting to the left.

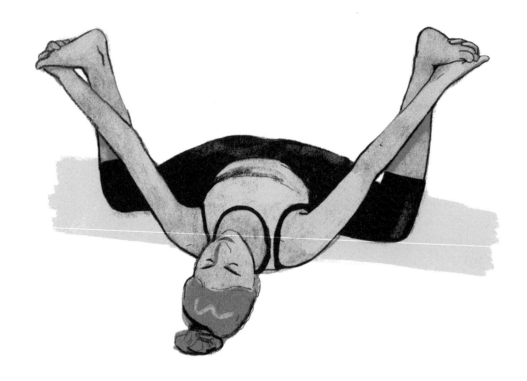

Happy Baby Pose

Ananda Balasana

The name of this pose says it all. This simple position feels so good that it will make you smile as you roll around on the ground. It gently but deeply stretches the hips and groins, and by lengthening the spine, it balances out the nervous system and calms the mind.

QUALITY Calming   **EFFECT** Balance, flexibility   **PROPS** None   **GAZE** Up

1   Begin lying on your back. If your spine is uncomfortable, place a thin blanket under your back. Draw your knees in to your chest. Separate your knees and feet wide and lift them up toward the sky, keeping your knees bent.

2   Grab the outer edges of your feet with your hands and gently pull your knees toward your armpits. Stack your ankles over your knees, bringing the shins perpendicular to the ground.

3   Lengthen your tailbone down and draw your shoulders back toward the ground.

4   Rock from side to side, gently massaging your lower back and spine.

5   Stay here for 5 to 10 breaths. Bring your knees closer to the ground with each exhale.

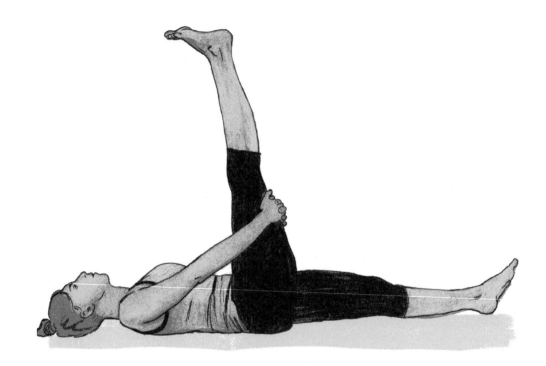

Supine One-Leg Stretch Pose

Supta Padangusthasana

This pose is an excellent way to start stretching and lengthening your hamstrings in preparation for the more intense standing and seated forward bends that call for hamstring flexibility. It also releases the lower back, and is great to practice after running, sitting at a desk, or as a transition pose from a backbend to forward bending. Make sure you have a strap handy.

QUALITY Calming **EFFECT** Flexibility, tranquility **PROPS** Strap **GAZE** Forward

1 Begin by lying on your back. Hug your right knee into your chest with your left leg long on the ground and flex your feet.

2 Draw your shoulders down toward the ground and away from your ears to lengthen the back of your neck and open your chest.

3 Place your strap around your foot or interlace your hands around the back of your right thigh, and lengthen your right leg straight up to the sky, flexing your foot and keeping your whole back on the ground.

4 Keep pressing your left leg and whole back body actively into the ground as you draw your right leg closer toward your head with each exhale.

5 Stay here for 8 to 10 breaths. Use your breath and gravity, rather than force, to deepen into the pose.

6 When you're ready to release the stretch, hug both knees into your chest and switch legs.

SEATED TWISTS AND FORWARD BENDS

These poses are detoxifying and purifying, and are meant to be practiced toward the end of your routine when the body is warmed up and the mind is quiet. This is the time when mind and body are more receptive to the longer holds and introspection. Forward bends slow down the practice and help you turn within, while twists help wring out tension from the musculoskeletal system and activate the internal organs responsible for detoxification. The poses are also meant to liberate you from your past, opening up the back body so you can move forward in life.

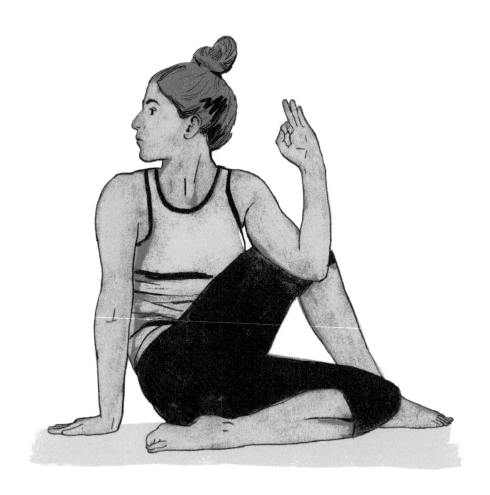

Seated Spinal Twist Pose

Ardha Matsyendrasana

One of the most beneficial of the cleansing twists, this pose has the sensation of wringing out a sponge as you twist. Microcirculation is increased to the discs within the spine. The nervous system is relaxed and the mind calmed. Twisting from the navel is believed to stoke the digestive fire, assisting in digestion and metabolism. It helps to reduce fatigue, back pain, tension, and sciatica and stimulates the kidneys and liver.

QUALITY Energizing, grounding   **EFFECT** Cleansing, invigoration, tranquility
PROPS Blanket   **GAZE** Back and down

1   Begin by sitting on your mat with your legs crossed. Place the sole of your right foot on the ground with your knee pointing up toward the sky, keeping the left leg open on the mat. Sit up tall, hugging your right shin into your chest.

2   Now cross your right leg over your left. Place the sole of your right foot outside your left thigh and your left foot on the outside edge of your right buttock.

3   Inhale while you lift your arms up above your head and exhale while you twist to the right, placing your left elbow on the outside your right knee, index finger and thumb together, and your right fingertips on the ground behind you. Look back behind your right shoulder.

4   Inhale to lengthen your spine and exhale to twist deeper, spiraling from your center. Draw your right hip down and reach the crown of your head up toward the sky.

5   Tuck your chin in slightly to lengthen the back of your neck and roll your shoulders back to lift your chest.

6   Stay here for 5 to 8 breaths. When you're ready to release, do a counter twist to the left, releasing your head toward the ground on the outside of your left hip to flood the right side of your body with prana, or life force, and to flush out the internal organs.

7   Repeat on the left side.

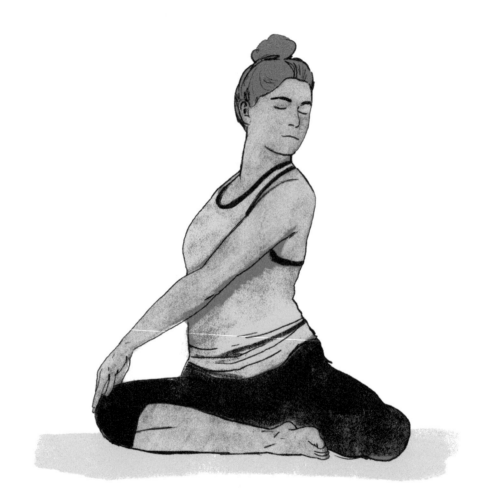

Sage Twist Pose

Bharadvajasana

This is another seated twist that can be held for a longer period of time and is a good preparation for seated meditation. It balances and calms the mind and also stretches the hips, spine, and shoulders, expanding the lungs and lengthening the spine and neck. This asana has all of the cleansing properties of twists and will leave you feeling refreshed and peaceful.

QUALITY Calming, energizing, grounding   EFFECT Cleansing, flexibility, stability
PROPS Blanket   GAZE Down and inward

1   Begin in a seated position with your legs crossed. Place the sole of your left foot on the ground and reach for your left ankle. Slide the top of this ankle down and back and place the top of your foot on the ground. Adjust yourself so that your heel is outside your left hip and your thigh is pointing forward. This puts you into half of a Hero's Pose (page 143).

2   Roll your right thigh and hip open as you draw your left inner thigh down and roll onto your right hip slightly.

3   Inhale your arms up toward the sky and twist to the right as you exhale, placing your right fingertips to the ground behind you and your left hand on your right knee.

4   Twist all the way to the right. Lift your chest by wrapping your shoulder blades around your upper spine and drawing your shoulders down.

5   Keep your chest open and twisting to the right, but look past your left shoulder and down to lengthen the right side of your neck.

6   Stay here for 5 to 8 breaths, inhaling to lift your chest and lengthen your spine, and exhaling to ground your hips and twist deeper from the navel.

7   When you're ready to release, do a counter twist to the left, and then switch legs.

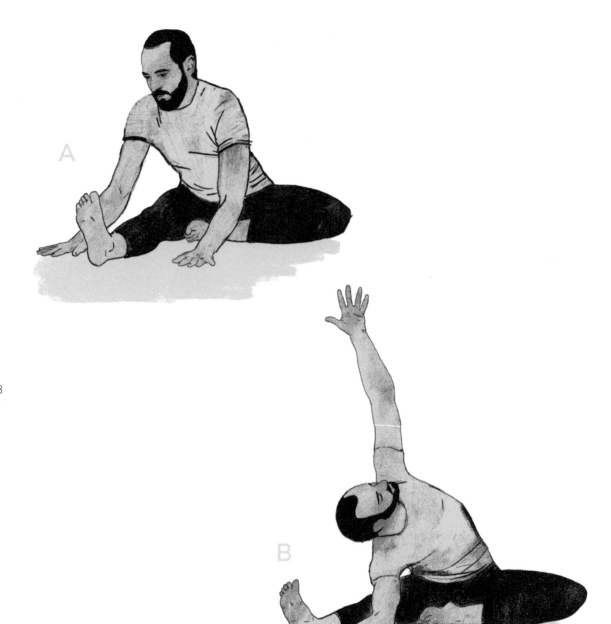

One-Leg Side Stretch Pose

Parivrtta Janu Sirsasana

Combining this pose with One-Leg Forward Bend calms the mind and reduces stress along with stretching the hamstrings and opening the hips.

QUALITY Calming, grounding   EFFECT Cleansing, flexibility, tension relief
PROPS Strap, blanket   GAZE Forward and inward

1 Begin in a seated position with your legs in front of you. Bend your left knee so your calf is close to your thigh. Place the sole of your left foot on the ground along the inside of your right leg.

2 Slide your left foot onto your inner right thigh and release your knee toward the ground (A). If your knee is very elevated, place a block under the knee for support or sit on the edge of a blanket to elevate your hips and release the spine.

3 Place your right hand on the ground outside your left hip and inhale as you lift your left arm up toward the sky, putting a slight bend in your right knee. Twist to the left and reach for the outside of your right foot with your right hand, drawing your right ribs down. Fold over your right leg with your forehead reaching toward your right knee.

4 Once you're centered over your right leg, reach for the inside of your right foot with your right hand. Inhale to stretch your chest forward and flex your right foot, drawing your shoulders back to lengthen your spine, and exhale to fold deeper over your leg.

5 Stay here for 5 to 8 breaths, releasing tension from your hamstrings and lower back with each exhale.

6 To move on to One-Leg Side Stretch, place your right forearm on the inside of your right shin and open your left knee and hip a little to twist open your chest. Reach your left arm up to the sky and over your ear, toward your right foot, lengthening the left side of your body (B).

7 Keep your chin in toward your chest to lengthen the back of your neck, and take your gaze to your right fingertips.

8 Root down into your left hip and hold for up to 5 breaths, stretching deeper on the exhales.

9 Exhale into the hips and raise your head. Place your left hand behind you, lift your hips to arch your back, and then switch legs.

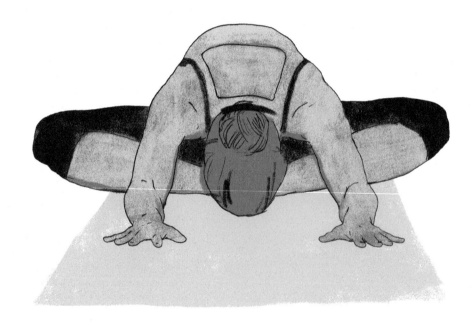

Bound Angle Pose

Baddha Konasana

This pose can be quite challenging at first for Westerners, since we tend to sit in chairs and cars. With a little practice and patience, you'll soon find yourself easing into the position, which increases flexibility in the hips, groins, knees, and inner thighs, and removes tension from the pelvis and reproductive organs. Both a forward bend and a hip opener, this pose is believed to help with menstrual discomfort, prostate health, hormonal imbalances, and preparation for childbirth.

QUALITY Calming, grounding   EFFECT Cleansing, flexibility, tranquility
PROPS Blocks, blanket   GAZE Inward

1 Begin in a seated position with your knees bent and the soles of your feet on the ground a few inches in front of you. Sit up tall and hug your knees into your chest.

2 Open your knees out to the sides toward the ground and draw the soles of your feet together. If your knees are very elevated, place a block under each knee or a blanket under your sit bones to elevate your hips and release your pelvis.

3 Wrap your hands around your feet and continue to sit up tall, lengthening your spine and drawing your shoulders down and back to lift your chest as your hips sink into the ground.

4 Begin to hinge forward from your hips, drawing your elbows back by your sides to extend forward with your chest and heart. Lengthen your spine as you keep rooting back thorough your hips, and fold forward as far as you can go, reaching your head toward the ground. You can place another block under your head to fully support the pose.

5 Stay here for 5 to 10 breaths. Relax and breathe into the pose instead of forcing or pushing it. Place a block under your head if you need it.

6 To come out of the pose, walk your hands back to lift yourself up to sit and draw your legs together, giving them a little shake before moving on to your next pose.

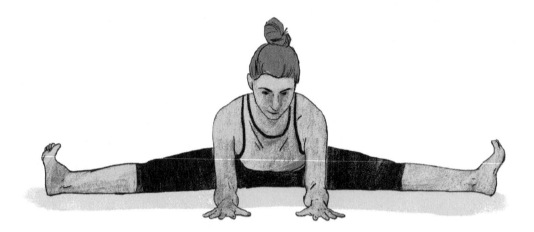

Straddle Forward Bend Pose

Upavistha Konasana

This pose is another simple one with infinite benefits to the body and mind, but it takes a lot of practice and surrender. Practice this one slowly. Each time, hold for a bit longer to stretch the legs, hamstrings, hips, and spine, using the breath to deepen into the pose.

QUALITY Calming, grounding   EFFECT Cleansing, flexibility, tranquility
PROPS Block, blanket   GAZE Inward

1   Begin in a seated position with your legs crossed. Place a folded blanket under the edge of your sit bones. Straighten your legs and open them to the sides, one at a time, as wide as they will go.

2   Sit up tall with your hands behind you to lengthen your spine. Open your chest by drawing your shoulders down and away from your ears.

3   Flex your feet and bend your knees a bit to actively roll your thighs out from your hips. Walk your hands forward in front of you between your legs as you press back with your hips.

4   Keep walking your hands forward as far as they will go, reaching your chest toward the ground. Place your forearms on the ground or on blocks. Press your chest forward, continuing to draw your shoulders back to open your chest and lengthen your spine.

5   Stay here for 5 to 8 breaths, lengthening your legs and spine with every exhale. Next, reach for your feet with your hands and release deeper into the pose for another 5 to 8 breaths.

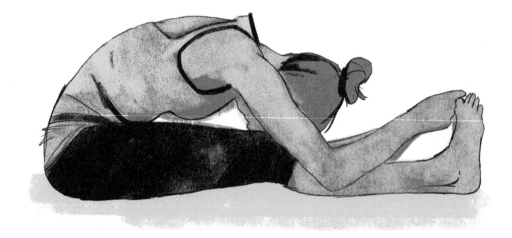

Full Forward Bend Pose

Paschimottanasana

This pose is another of deep surrender, so make sure you're warmed up through Sun Salutations (page 199) and standing poses so you can release deeply in to the pose and receive its many benefits. This pose stretches the entire back body. It's also thought to stimulate the internal organs, promoting digestion and detoxification, relieving anxiety and stress, and helping with menstrual discomfort and hormonal imbalances.

QUALITY Calming, grounding   **EFFECT** Cleansing, flexibility, tranquility
PROPS Blanket, strap   **GAZE** Inward

1 Begin in a seated position on the ground with a folded blanket under the edge of your sit bones and your legs together, stretched out in front of you.

2 Place your hands behind you to sit up tall, lengthening your spine. Open your chest by drawing your shoulders back and away from your ears. Flex your feet to activate your legs.

3 Bend your knees slightly and inhale while raising your arms up. Exhale and fold forward over your legs, hinging at the hips.

4 Keeping your knees bent, reach for the outer edges of your feet and draw your chest forward and shoulders back, lengthening your spine and deeply contracting your abdomen. This stokes the digestive fire and promotes purification.

5 Modification: If your hands don't reach your feet, place a strap around your feet and hold it tightly with both hands while extending your spine forward.

6 Draw your chin toward your chest and turn your gaze within. Stay here for 8 to 10 breaths.

7 When you're ready, root down into your sit bones to rise up.

RESTORATIVE AND RELAXATION POSES

Relaxation is just as much of a skill, practice, and art as some of the more complicated and dynamic poses in yoga. Like using and discovering new muscles, relaxation through restorative and resting poses can be quite challenging, especially if you're stressed out or agitated. They are wonderful to practice at the end of a full practice but can be done anytime on their own to help you reconnect with your inner peace. These poses are generally held from 5 to 10 minutes, and are often supported by props such as blankets, bolsters, and eye pillows to deepen your relaxation.

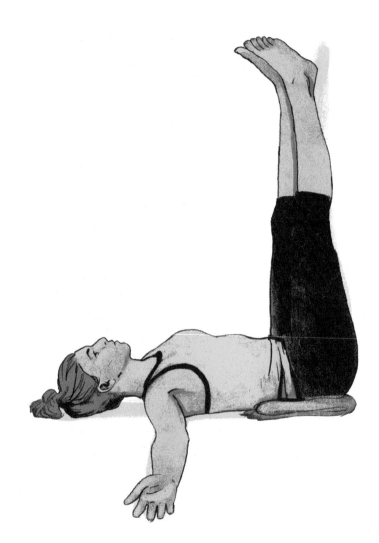

Legs Up the Wall Pose

Viparita Karani

This is yoga's magical pose to reboot and rejuvenate your whole body, mind, and spirit! As an inversion, it is meant to defy aging. It relieves your legs, feet, spine, and nervous system, bringing the body into a state of deep relaxation and renewal. You can practice this pose anytime to receive all of its incredible benefits. Among other things, it strengthens the immune system, calms the nervous system, and balances the digestive and elimination systems.

QUALITY Calming   **EFFECT** Cleansing, relaxation, and tranquility
PROPS Blanket or block   **GAZE** Inward

1   Slide the top of your mat against a wall and bring a folded blanket with you. Lie down on your back and scoot your hips as close to the wall as you can. Bend your knees and place your feet on the wall.

2   Press your feet into the wall to lift up your hips and slide a folded blanket or block under your sacrum or lower back to elevate your heart. You may need to move around and adjust the lift a bit until you're comfortable. Then, place your hands on your belly and breathe slowly and deeply. You can also lift your arms over your head to release your shoulders and neck.

3   If you have an eye pillow, place it over your eyes to release mental tension and melt away stress. This posture can be held for 5 to 10 minutes, depending on how much time you have. You can also bend your knees and place the soles of your feet together, opening your hips and knees toward the wall.

4   When you're ready to come out of this pose, bend your knees to lift your hips and remove the support under you. As you release your hips back down to the ground, hug your knees into your chest and breathe into your lower back. Roll over to your right side to come up to sit.

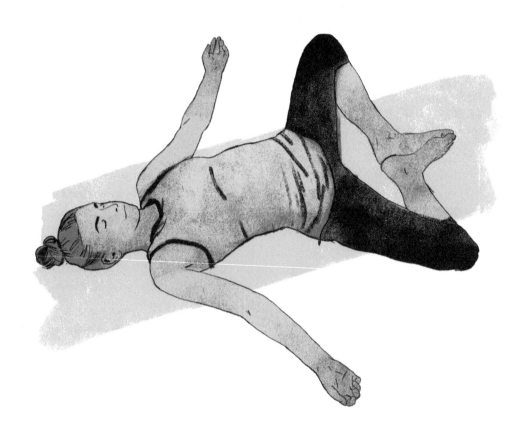

Goddess Pose

Utkata Konasana

This restorative pose is like a little vacation that relaxes the mind, body, and spirit. Practice the pose anytime to receive its believed health benefits, including lowered blood pressure and reduced muscle tension, headaches, fatigue, stress, and insomnia. In addition, this pose encourages relaxation of the abdominal muscles, and is thought to relieve irritable bowel syndrome and aid in reproductive health. It's a deep hip opener that stretches the groins and inner thighs and opens the chest, lungs, and heart. Make sure you have two blocks handy.

QUALITY Calming   **EFFECT** Tranquility, relaxation, rejuvenation   **PROPS** Blocks   **GAZE** Internal

1 Begin in a seated position. Bend your knees and draw your heels in toward your pelvis. Press the soles of your feet together and let your knees drop open to both sides. If needed, place a block under each knee for full support. Lean back and bring your elbows to the ground, lowering your back all the way to the ground.

2 Feel free to adjust your position so your spine lowers to the ground. Draw your shoulder blades together to relax your shoulders and let your arms rest by your sides with your palms facing up.

3 Close your eyes and, if you have one, place an eye pillow over your eyes to deepen the restorative effects of the pose. Place your hands on your belly for a few deep Supine Belly Breaths (page 213). Let your awareness draw within, and lower your body farther into the ground with each exhale.

4 Stay here for 3 to 10 minutes. When you're ready, slowly draw your knees into your chest to release your back before rolling onto your right side to come up to sit.

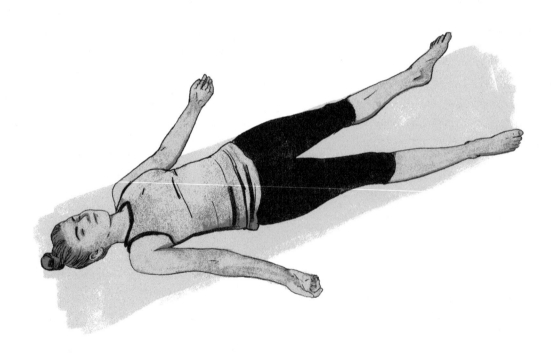

Deep Relaxation Pose

Savasana

Welcome to the most important and most challenging pose of yoga: Deep Relaxation, or savasana, which means "corpse" in Sanskrit. Although it may seem easy to lie down and do nothing, this pose is meant to be a practice of complete surrender and letting go. Lying completely still and resting your fidgety body and racing mind is no small task. In this pose, you'll find that your worries and stress seem to melt away. This pose is known for its deeply therapeutic and restorative benefits. It calms the nerves, relieves insomnia, anxiety, and fatigue, and increases energy, concentration, and memory. Playing soothing instrumental music is a nice way to assist you in fully letting go in this pose.

QUALITY Calming **EFFECT** Relaxation, rejuvenation, tranquility
PROPS Blanket, eye pillow (optional) **GAZE** Internal

1 Make sure you are warm and comfortable. Begin in a seated position with your legs in front of you, and place a rolled blanket or bolster under your knees. Begin to recline onto your back with your arms at your sides. If your neck is uncomfortable, place a blanket under your head. Place an eye pillow over your eyes, if you have one.

2 Allow your arms to rest at your sides about 6 inches away from your body with your palms up, and let your feet roll open to the sides.

3 Close your eyes and bring your awareness to your natural breath. With each exhale, surrender the weight of your body deeper to the force of gravity.

4 From your feet to your head, consciously release every part of your body. Relax all the muscles in your face. Completely surrender to silence and peace, and explore your inner world by drawing all your senses inward.

5 Stay here for 5 to 20 minutes. When you're ready, slowly draw your awareness back to your breath and then your body by moving your fingers and toes and stretching your arms above your head.

6 Hug your knees into your chest, and roll to your right side in a fetal position. Rest here as a transition pose, before you make your way up to sit, and reenter your life embodying peace and love, ready to share it with all.

WARM-UPS

In yoga philosophy, the safe sequencing of a class or practice is referred to as vinyasa karma, *meaning "wise progression" or "step by step," so that each pose is practiced as a preparation for the next. It starts with contemplation, followed by a well-constructed sequence based on what the body needs, and then moves toward a climax at the top of the practice that closes with a cooldown in preparation for a final meditation and relaxation. Each pose has its own health benefits and powerful effects, so proper consideration of how one practices, as well as what one practices, is one of yoga's greatest teachings.*

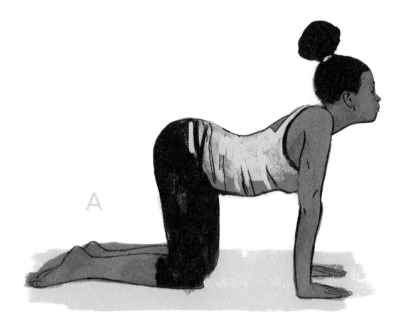

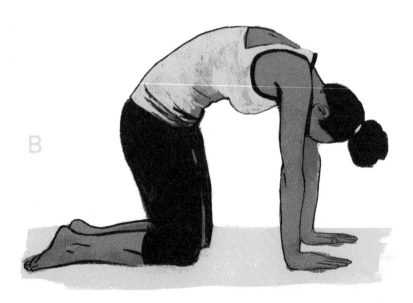

Cat-Cow Pose

Marjaryasana-Bitilasana

This simple exercise warms up, massages, and loosens the whole spine. It calms and soothes the mind, helping you to begin coordinating your movements with the rhythm of your breath.

QUALITY Calming **EFFECT** Relaxation, tranquility **PROPS** None **GAZE** Up and inward

1   Begin in Child's Pose (page 35). Take 5 long deep full breaths here, slowing your breaths to a 4-count inhale and a 4-count exhale.

2   On the next inhale, rise up to your hands and knees, with your hands directly under your shoulders and your knees under your hips and with a long, neutral spine.

3   As you inhale, lift your tailbone and drop your belly as you look up, drooping your spine into Cow Pose (A). As you exhale, draw your tailbone in and round your spine, dropping your chin toward your chest as you pull your belly in and arch your spine into Cat Pose (B).

4   Lengthen the breath to about 3 counts per inhale and 3 counts per exhale, coordinating your movements with your breath about 8 to 10 times. Feel free to move your hips from side to side and circle your head to relieve any tension in your lower back and neck. When you're done, move your hips back to your heels and into Child's Pose.

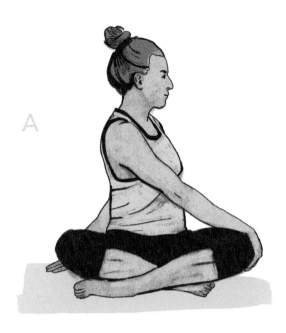

A

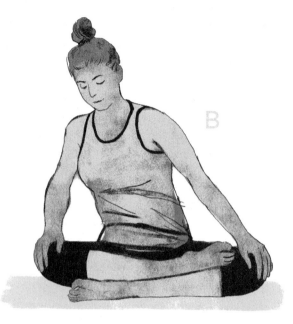

B

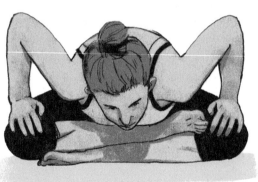

C

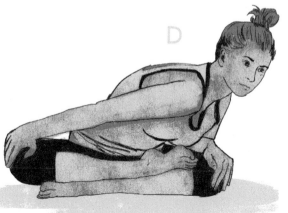

D

Cleansing Circles and Twists

This invigorating warm-up cleanses the internal organs and removes fatigue and stiffness from the hips, spine, and shoulders.

QUALITY Energizing EFFECT Cleansing PROPS Block GAZE Different directions

1 Begin in a seated position with your knees bent and your legs crossed. As you inhale, raise your arms above your head, looking up. As you exhale, rotate your chest to the left and place your left hand behind you on the ground or on a block and your right hand to your left knee (A). Sit up tall as you breathe into your belly. As you exhale, twist from your navel, drawing it in and up, and look past your left shoulder. Stay here for 3 breaths, sitting up taller on each inhale, and twisting and relaxing the shoulders away from the ears on each exhale.

2 After 3 breaths, reach your left arm up and over your head, leaning to the right for a side stretch. Fold forward with your left hand to your right knee, and breathe into the hips and back of body. Inhale and rise up with your right arm under your left knee and arch your back, breathing into the back of your ribs. Circle your arms back up above your head, and exhale and twist to the right, with your left hand on your right knee and right hand behind you on the ground. Stay here for 3 breaths.

3 Come back to the center with your hands on your knees. Bend forward and to the right to begin making big wide circles with your spine (B). As you inhale, circle the chest forward, (C), and as you exhale, rotate it back (D), rounding your spine with your chin tucked toward your chest. Circle 9 times to the right, and then reverse and circle 9 times to the left. After the last rotation, raise your arms up and place both hands behind you and your feet on the ground in front of you with bent knees. Inhale your hips up and exhale strongly though your mouth, sticking out your tongue for Lion's Breath (see Warrior Goddess, page 73). Do this 3 times, and return your hips to your seated position.

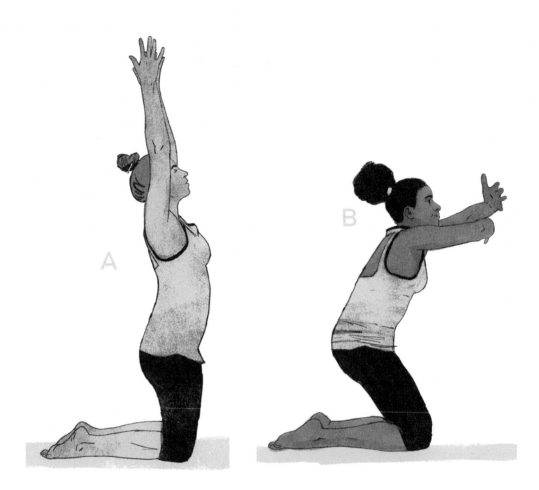

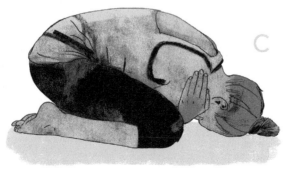

Tibetan Sun Salutation

Surya Namaskara

This warm-up is a mini Sun Salutation (page 199) that gently wakes up the body and mind, coordinating the breath with movement. It is a full body breathing practice and perfect to do first thing in the morning—the effects are better than a cup of coffee!

QUALITY Energizing, calming, grounding   **EFFECT** Cleansing, rejuvenation
PROPS Blanket   **GAZE** Up and inward

1   Begin in Child's Pose (page 35). On your next inhale, rise up onto your shins, lifting your hips off your heels as you circle your arms above you (A), and look up. As you exhale, hold on to opposite elbows (B), draw your forearms into your belly, and fold over your arms, bowing your head to the earth (C). Empty all your breath out and then rise up while inhaling, circling your arms above you, and exhale to fold forward again.

2   Repeat 3 times, keeping your breath long, deep, and slow. Then, feel free to pick up the pace to make the motion more dynamic, especially if you need extra energy. Repeat 8 or 9 more times. Make sure to slow it down again before returning to Child's Pose.

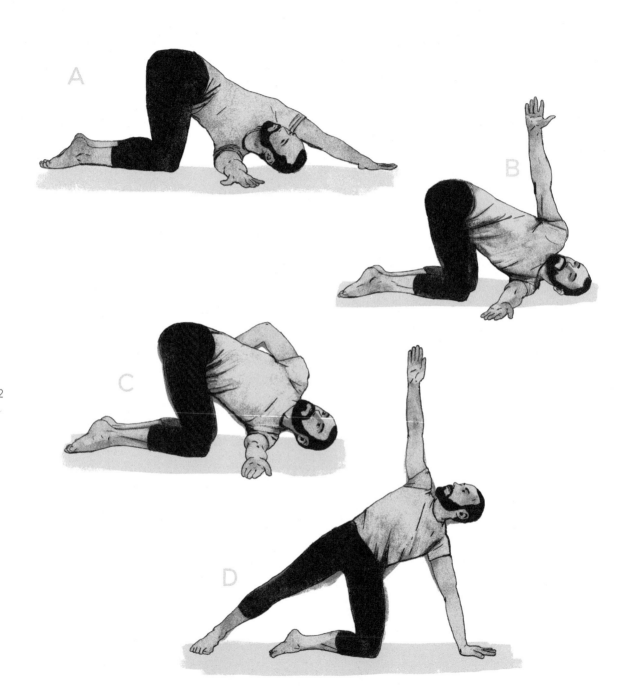

Thread the Needle Pose

Sucirandhrasana

This warm-up opens the shoulders and relieves stiffness in the neck. It's the perfect stretch after work or a long day. I also love to practice this warm-up first thing in the morning as a simple wake-up stretch. It helps me to get into my body and breath and prepares me for anything I have to do next.

QUALITY Grounding   **EFFECT** Flexibility, stability, strength   **PROPS** Blanket   **GAZE** Forward and up

1   Begin on your hands and knees, placing your hands directly under your shoulders and knees under your hips. Shift your left hand to the center of your mat, and inhale your right arm up to the sky

2   Turn and twist your gaze and your chest open to the right. As you exhale, thread your right arm under your left, releasing the right shoulder and ear to the ground. Press deeply into the left hand to release any pressure in the neck. You can lengthen your left arm forward (A), reach it up into the sky (B), or eventually snake it behind you to open your left shoulder (C). Take 3 long breaths here, dissolving the tension from your shoulders into the ground.

3   On your next inhale, breathe the right arm up to the sky and stretch the right leg back. Seal your right heel to the ground and keep your left shin rooted with your knee under your hip, in a Supported Side Incline Plank Pose (D). Open the whole right side of your body, stretching your right arm over your head and arching your back slightly. Take 3 deep breaths here, stretching open on each exhale.

4   Shift back into Child's Pose (page 35), and come back onto your hands and knees before doing Thread the Needle on the left side.

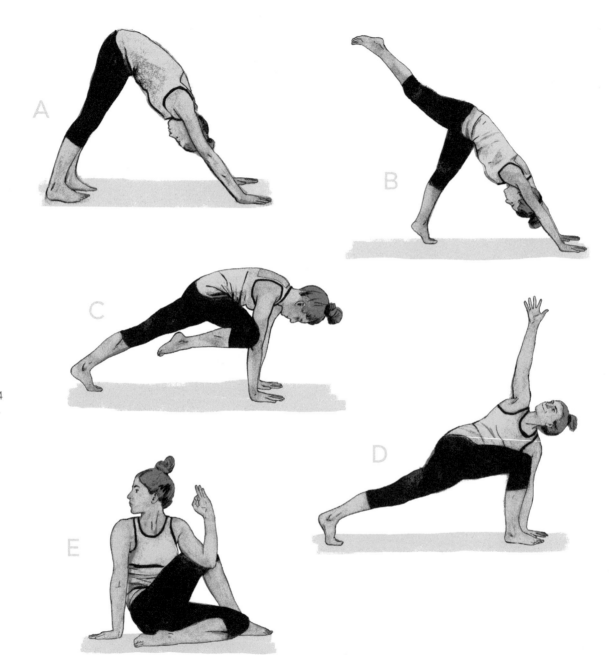

Stoke the Fire Pose

This warm-up is for when you could use extra lift and power in your practice to feel strong, warm, and confident all day. The focus on breath, twisting, and core work heats up and energizes the body and wakes up the mind. This pose is perfect during the winter months when we are a little more sluggish.

QUALITY Energizing **EFFECT** Alertness, focus, heat, invigoration, strength
PROPS Block and blanket **GAZE** Forward and Up

1 Start in a seated position with your legs crossed or sitting on your shins. Starting with Bellows Breath (page 219), place your hands on your belly and take 3 deep belly breaths, moving the navel away from the spine on the inhale and drawing it in on the exhale. After breath 3, begin pumping the navel in and out, breathing through your nose. This is called Bellows Breath because it mimics a bellows stoking a fire. Repeat 20 times and hold the last breath out. Drop your chin to your chest and slowly inhale and exhale.

2 Come onto your hands and knees and make your way to Downward-Facing Dog (A). Stay here for 3 breaths, pressing your hands into the ground and lengthening your spine as you stretch the backs of your legs.

3 As you inhale, reach your right leg into the sky (B). As you exhale, bend your right knee and draw it to your left elbow, and hold for 1 breath. Inhale while you reach your right leg back up into the sky, and exhale while you bring your right leg to the outside of your right elbow (C), and hold for 1 breath. Inhale while you reach your right leg up to the sky again, and this time draw your right knee toward your nose and hold for 1 breath, then release your foot down between your hands into a lunge.

4 On your next inhale, reach your right arm to the sky into a Lunge Twist (D). Breathe in to open your chest and exhale to twist from your core. Stay here for 2 breaths, then tuck your left knee behind your right ankle and sit down in a Seated Spinal Twist (E). Stay here for 2 breaths, twisting deeper with each exhale.

continued >

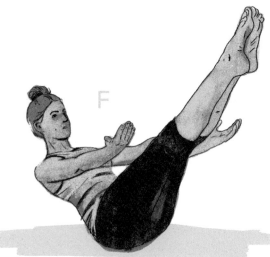

F

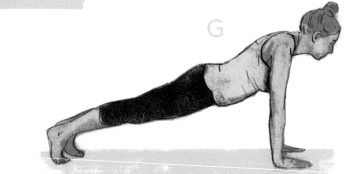

G

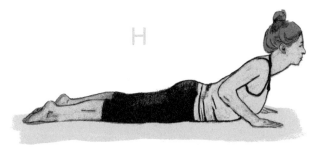

H

5 Next, place both hands behind you and both feet in front of you. Lift your hips up to the sky and exhale through your mouth. Return your hips to the ground and hug your knees into your chest before coming into Boat Pose (F), straightening out your legs and reaching them up to the sky. Stay here for 3 breaths, reaching your arms forward, before crossing your ankles and returning to Downward-Facing Dog.

6 As you inhale, move forward into a Plank Pose (G), and hold for 3 breaths.

7 See if you can stay lifted in your navel as you bend your arms and lower yourself all the way down to the ground. Point your toes and inhale to lift your head, shoulders, and chest off the ground into Baby Cobra (H).

8 Press deeply into your hands and lift yourself back into Downward-Facing Dog as you exhale. Repeat the sequence on the left side. End with Downward-Facing Dog before releasing your knees to the ground and your hips to your heels for Child's Pose.

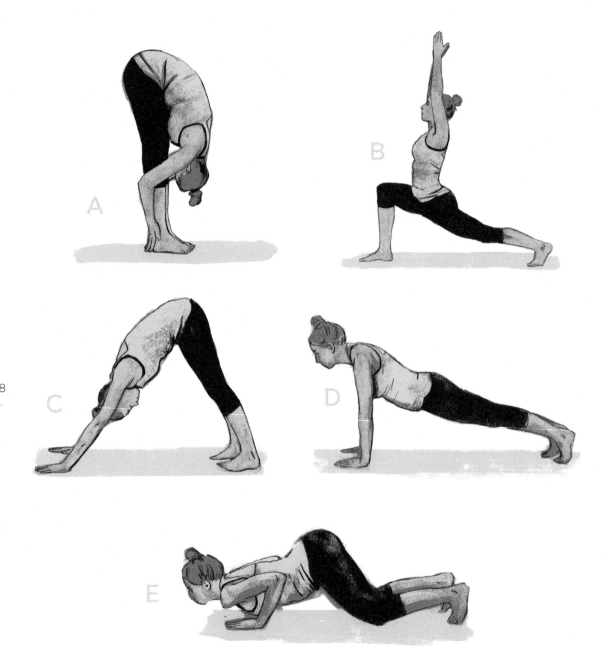

Full Sun Salutation

Surya Namasakara

This warm-up is an ode to the sun, a moving mantra and meditation, as well as a full breathing practice. It is practiced with 1 breath per movement and warms up the body and quiets the mind in preparation for the day or the rest of your practice. You can practice this sequence in a slow, soothing rhythm or a faster, more dynamic one.

QUALITY Energizing, calming, grounding   **EFFECT** Flexibility, heat, concentration, strength
PROPS Blocks   **GAZE** Different directions as you move

1 Begin in Mountain Pose (page 49) with your hands at your heart as if in prayer. Face east, if possible, to greet the sun. Take a moment to give gratitude for something or someone in your life.

2 Inhale, and circle your arms up above you. As you exhale, look up and draw the prayer down through your heart and to the ground in gratitude, and move into a Standing Forward Bend (A).

3 As you inhale, move your right leg back into a High Lunge (B) while looking up, then exhale as you move into Down-ward-Facing Dog (C).

4 As you inhale, move like a wave into Plank Pose (D), and exhale to Knees, Chest, Chin (E).

continued >

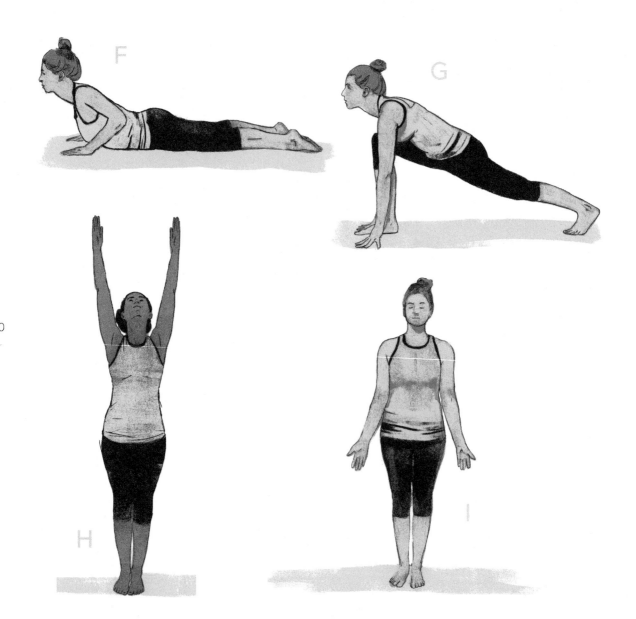

5 Inhale as you push yourself up to Baby Cobra (F), and exhale while you move back to Downward-Facing Dog.

6 Inhale while moving your right leg up and exhale as you plant your foot between your hands into Low Lunge (G). Inhale as you look up, lifting your face into the light, and exhale as you move into Standing Forward Bend. Inhale as you rise up like the sun in the sky (H), and exhale as you place your hands near your heart. Lower your arms by your side in Mountain Pose (I).

7 Repeat on the left side, stepping back with the left leg. Practice 1 to 3 rounds altogether.

COOLDOWN POSES

Cooldowns are just as essential as warm-ups. Held for longer, these poses slow everything down and prepare the body and mind for meditation and relaxation. They're great on their own but better when the body is warmed up. These poses are best to do when the mind is already quiet and can focus on relaxing or on holding longer restorative poses. Make sure to leave yourself plenty of time for these essential poses in your practice.

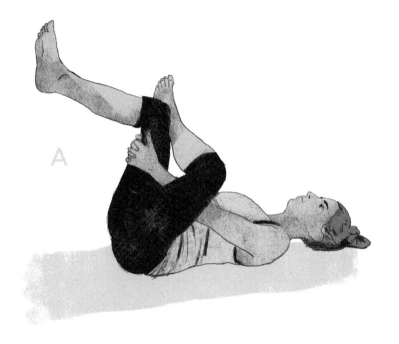

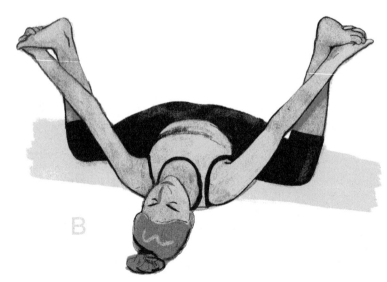

Supine Pigeon Pose

Supta Kapotasana

King Pigeon (page 153) is one of the most cooling, soothing, and restorative poses to end almost any practice. Variations on this pose are great if you need to cool down after a dynamic practice or wrap up a more restorative practice. Supine Pigeon is a gentler version.

QUALITY Calming **EFFECT** Flexibility, stress relief **Prop** Blanket, strap
GAZE Inward and forward

1 Begin by lying on your back with your knees bent. Cross your left ankle over your right knee and rotate your hip open, flexing your foot to protect your knee.

2 Take a few breaths here and then slowly begin to wrap your arms around your right thigh, pulling your left shin closer to your chest with each exhale (A). Inhale to release a little and exhale to hug your shin in, breathing into your hips and back to relieve any tightness or strain.

3 After 8 to 10 breaths, lengthen your right leg and walk your hands up your leg toward your ankle to stretch the right hamstring and left hip. Keep pressing your back and shoulders into the ground and breathe until you are ready to come out of the position.

4 Hug both knees into your chest and repeat on the right side, crossing the right ankle over the left knee. When you're finished with the right side, reach for the outside edges of both feet and draw your knees toward your armpits for Happy Baby (B), a double hip stretch.

5 Finish by releasing your body into Deep Relaxation Pose (page 183) for a few minutes, allowing your body to completely relax before coming up to sit.

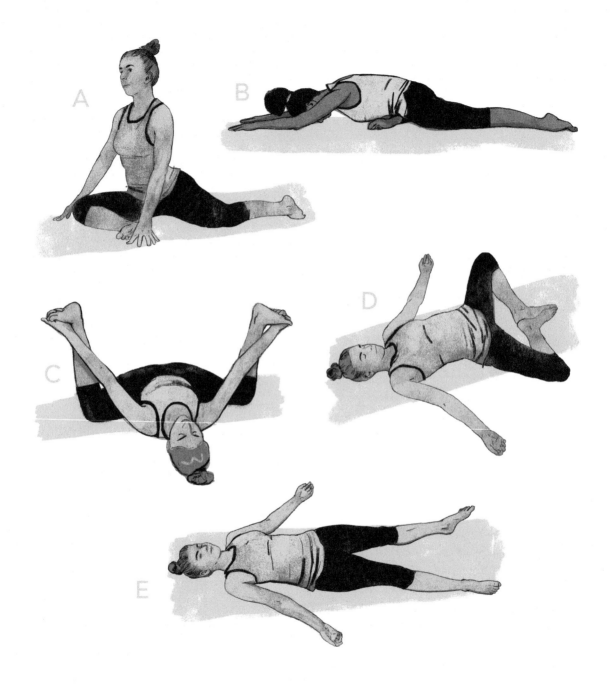

Seated and Resting Pigeon

Eka Pada Kapotasana

Seated and Resting Pigeon are deeply grounding, restful, and soothing after a dynamic practice or any time you need to chill out.

QUALITY Calming, grounding   **EFFECT** Flexibility, stress relief
Prop Blanket, 2 blocks   **GAZE** Forward

1   Begin in Downward-Facing Dog (page 37).

2   Raise your right leg into the sky and bend your knee to peel open your right hip, drawing your right heel toward your left sit bone. Inhale to stretch your leg long behind you. Exhale to draw your shin forward, parallel with the top of your mat. Place a folded blanket under your right hip, if needed.

3   Tuck your left toes under and walk your hands back to lengthen your spine. Make sure your hips are centered, with the right hip drawing back and the left hip drawing forward into a Seated Pigeon (A). Slowly begin to walk your hands forward into Resting Pigeon (B), lying your chest toward the ground. Stay still and take at least 8 to 10 breaths.

4   Walk both of your hands under your shoulders, lift your chest, and step back into Downward-Facing Dog.

5   Pedal your feet to relieve your legs, and then repeat on the left side, lifting your left leg up and bending your knee to open your hip before drawing it forward toward the top of your mat into Seated Pigeon Pose.

6   Release your knees to the ground into Child's Pose (page 35). Take 3 to 5 breaths here, then rise up onto your shins and lower down onto your back for Happy Baby Pose (C). Stay here for 5 breaths.

7   Bend your knees and place the soles of your feet together, opening your hips into Goddess Pose (D). Place the blocks under your knees for support. Place one hand on your belly and one on your heart. Breathe into your heart and chest, through your belly and into your lower abdomen to further release the hips.

8   After 8 to 10 breaths like this, lengthen your legs out in front of you into Deep Relaxation Pose (E), allowing your body to release into the ground for 5 to 10 minutes. Slowly rise up to sit.

4

Breathing Practice

"Breathe. Let go. And remind yourself that this very moment is the only one you know you have for sure." —OPRAH WINFREY

Our breath plays an integral role in the functioning of our entire body and is also a reflection of our emotions and state of mind. Better breathing patterns make us more present and grounded, ready to take on whatever comes our way. When our breathing goes awry, we may find ourselves stressed, overwhelmed, and out of balance. The same is true in reverse: When we're happy and healthy, we tend to breathe easier. With conscious breathing, we can impact our inner world.

What Is Good Breathing?

Learning to consciously regulate our breath is one of the most powerful tools we can cultivate. It helps us control our emotions and let go. As we covered earlier in the book, yogic breathing practices are called *pranayama*, which means "to control or extend the breath." *Prana* is our "life force" and *ayama* means "to extend." With slow, regulated breathing, the quality of our lives improves dramatically.

When we are stressed, our breath becomes shallow. We breathe quickly and only fill up the top part of our lungs with oxygen. Our chest barely expands with each inhale, which triggers our fight-or-flight stress response.

In contrast, when we're fully relaxed and present, our breath becomes slower and deeper. This triggers our rest-and-digest response, which lowers our heart rate. With each inhale, our entire chest and belly expand, flooding us with oxygen. With each exhale, we fully contract all of these parts of the body, releasing carbon dioxide. In this manner, each full inhale nourishes every part of our being, while each complete exhale cleanses and releases toxins from the mind and body.

Why does all of this matter? Well, the average human being takes over 20,000 breaths a day. Each breath brings us the opportunity to positively affect our state of mind and benefit our overall health. When we talk about good breathing, we're talking about a conscious, slow, even, and deep breath that satisfies our need for oxygen while helping us maintain a calm and present state of mind. With conscious breathing comes conscious living. This is what we strive for in yoga.

Breathing Techniques

Yoga uses a variety of breathing or pranayama techniques to help facilitate different outcomes. Ujjayi breathing, which we discussed earlier (page 17), is one of the most common types of yogic breathing. Most often used during asana, it allows us to create a steady, even rhythmic breath, and to link our breath and movement. In this practice, every inhale is a movement that expands the chest, such as inhaling the arms up, and every exhale promotes a contraction, such as exhaling a forward bend. The inhale accompanies a movement (such as reaching the arms up), and the exhale accompanies another movement (such as moving into a forward bend). There are also slight pauses between breaths to help us experience stillness.

Long, deep breathing is used to calm the mind during meditation or anytime you're in a stressful situation. This breath focuses on expanding and contracting the belly to engage the diaphragm and create a slow, even breath with a slightly longer exhale. This allows for space to calm the nerves, quiet the mind, and let go.

When you're feeling sluggish, a bellows breath can be just what you need. This exercise pumps breath from the belly rapidly and simulates the effects of aerobic exercise, including increased metabolism, increased heart rate, and the release of serotonin to the brain.

Alternate nose breathing, where you use your thumb and pointer finger to alternately cover each nostril, is thought to align the left and right hemispheres of the brain and balance our emotional state.

All of these techniques can help you breathe better to live better.

Breathing Exercises

Although we are breathing all the time, *conscious* breathing techniques take a little time to master. Be patient and curious, and remember that with mastering your breath comes mastering your mind, mood, and movement. Here is one tip as you get started: Yoga masters believe that the exhalation is the most important part of the breath, since it makes space for the inhale. While it may feel counterintuitive, begin each breathing exercise with a deep exhale.

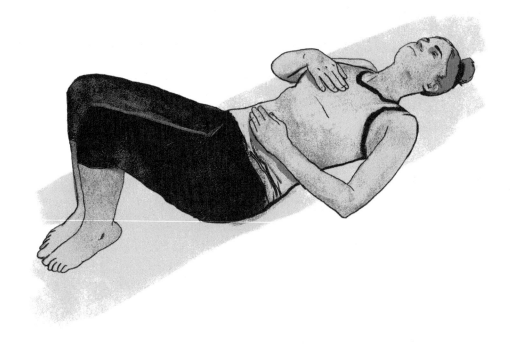

Simple Supine Belly Breath

The first step to cultivating better breathing habits is to practice tuning into your breath while lying down on your back. This way, your body is at ease and you can completely focus on the breath. I love to do this breathing practice in bed first thing in the morning and at night while unwinding from the day. It relieves anxiety and stress and floods the body with prana, leaving you refreshed and relaxed. Known as diaphragmatic breathing, it transforms shallow chest breathing to the body's natural relaxation response. It also melts away tension from the shoulders and neck caused by constricted breathing and massages the heart. Practice this breathing technique first before trying more complex breathing practices. The Simple Supine Belly Breath doesn't have to be done lying down; use this breath in all your practices and throughout the day.

1 Begin by lying down on your back on your mat. You can place a rolled-up blanket under your knees to release your lower back.

2 Place one hand on your belly and one on your chest, and begin to breathe in and out through your nose with your mouth closed, simply paying attention to your inhalations and exhalations.

3 As you inhale, breathe into your belly and feel it rise and expand away from the spine. As you exhale, draw in your ribs a little and empty out all of the air.

4 Now slow down your breath and inhale for a count of 4. Pause for 1 to 2 counts and then exhale for 6.

5 Practice this daily, for about 3 to 5 minutes in the morning and at night, or anytime you feel anxious, stressed, or tired. It's like a mini-retreat!

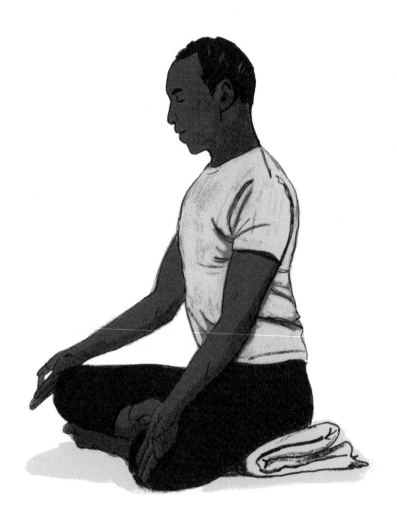

Warrior's Breath

Ujjayi Pranayama

Warrior's Breath, also translated as "victorious breath," is a technique used to quiet the mind and purify the body. In this breath, you'll constrict the throat to create an oceanic sound, making the breath more audible and easier to focus on during meditation and throughout your yoga practice. This Ujjayi breath energizes with its slight heating qualities and soothes with its hypnotic sound.

1   Begin in Easy Pose (page 15) or Hero's Pose (page 143) with padding under your hips, and root down and lengthen your spine. Draw your shoulders back to lift and open your chest, and place your hands on your thighs or your belly. Close your eyes and tune in to the natural rhythm of your breath with your mouth closed, breathing in and out though your nose.

2   Now drop your chin down slightly to lengthen the back of your neck but lift your gaze slightly up. As you breathe in, close the back of your throat slightly so when you breathe out, you can hear the sound of your breath. If you have trouble hearing this sound, open your mouth and exhale as if you are trying to fog up a mirror. Now close your mouth and see if you can create the

same sound again through your nose. This is the Ujjayi breath.

3   Once you've mastered the sound, tune in to the rhythm and try a 4-count breath, belly breathing for 3 to 5 minutes. You can practice this breathing technique whenever you need to feel victorious over your nerves or emotions in order to keep calm and present.

4   You can also move right into your asana practice, coordinating your movement with your breath as you flow from one pose to the next. This breath is great to do right before meditation, helping to calm your mind in preparation.

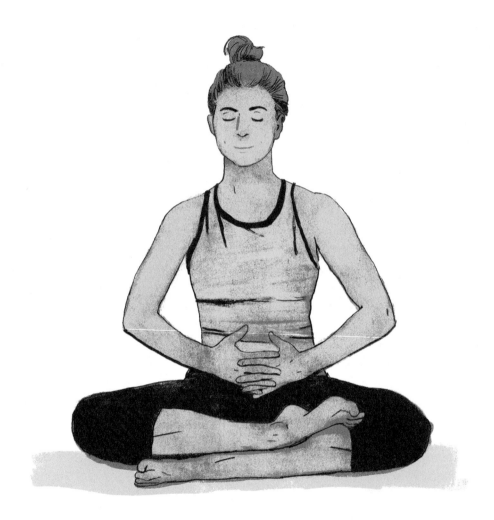

Cleansing Breath

Kapalbhati Pranayama

This practice is also called a kriya *or purifying practice. It's been known to clear out the respiratory system, sinuses, lungs, and mind, and to strengthen the abdominal muscles and diaphragm. The Sanskrit translates to "skull shining breath," referring to its ability to clear out darkness and stagnant energy from the mind and blockages from the body. This practice is great to do before your asana practice to wake you up and get you moving, before you start your day, or anytime you're feeling sluggish. Have some tissues nearby, as you may need to blow your nose!*

1 Begin in Easy Pose (page 15) or Hero's Pose (page 143) with padding under your hips, and root down and lengthen your spine. Draw your shoulders back to lift and open your chest, and place your hands on your thighs or your belly. Close your eyes and tune in to the natural rhythm of your breath with your mouth closed, breathing in and out though your nose.

2 Feel free to practice a few rounds of Warrior's Breath (page 215) to get started.

3 When you're ready, take a big breath into your belly and exhale strongly out through your nose for 1 count, drawing your navel back toward the spine, and pumping the breath out. Inhale passively and then exhale, pumping the breath out powerfully. Your focus should be on the exhale to purify the body and mind.

4 Start with 25 pumps with your hands on your lower belly to bring your awareness and breath into your navel. Slow down the breath when you near the end of your first round. Hold the last breath out with your chin toward your chest, retaining the exhale for as long as you can before returning to your natural breathing. Repeat once or twice and work up to 50 pumps per round.

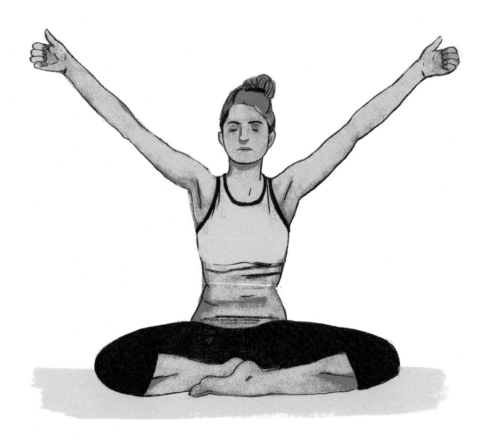

Bellows Breath (Breath of Fire)

Bhastrika Pranayama

As the name suggests, this breathing practice stokes the inner fire and burns away impurities in the body and mind as well as past karma. It's believed to purify the blood, awaken the solar plexus, and expand lung capacity as well as improve the digestive system and metabolism. It may also strengthen the nervous system and help regulate the endocrine system. The variation with your arms in a V, for victory, is called the "Ego Eradicator"; it calls on our will to go beyond the limitations of our thinking. It should only be practiced once you have mastered the other three breathing practices. If keeping your arms up is too challenging, place your hands on your belly to feel the pumping of your navel.

1 Begin in any comfortable seated position with your spine long and chest open.

2 Inhale your arms above your head and exhale them into a V shape on either side of your head. Draw your shoulders down but actively stretch your arms out.

3 Open your hands wide and bend your fingers into the top pads of your hands with your thumbs sticking straight out. Turn your upper arms out and roll your shoulders back.

4 Take a deep breath into your belly, filling it with as much air as you can, and exhale your navel strongly back toward your spine. Begin pumping the breath in and out in equal inhales and exhales, instead of only the exhales as we did in Cleansing Breath (page 217), like a bellows fanning a fire.

5 This breath is timed, so start with 1 minute, then 2, and work up to 5. Some yogis do this practice for 30 minutes continuously. Start out with a slow rhythm and eventually pick up the pace to a rapid one.

6 If your arms get tired, take them above your head with your thumbs touching and return them back down to a V. When your session is over, stretch your arms above you and hold the exhale with your chin in toward your chest. Then inhale deeply, slowly releasing your arms to your sides.

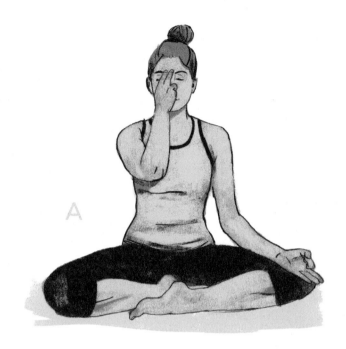

A

B

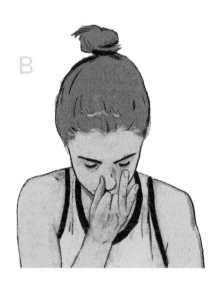

C

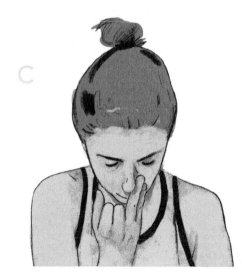

Alternate Nostril Breath

Nadi Shodhana Pranayama

This breathing technique should be a part of everyone's daily routine for health, happiness, and harmony. In yoga philosophy, there are two main channels of energy, solar and lunar, which come through each nostril and connect in the two hemispheres of the brain. This practice dissolves duality to bring about balance and bridge all opposites. It unblocks these two channels, which is essential, as yogis believe that any physical or mental disease originates through one or the other being blocked.

1 Begin in Easy Pose (page 15) or Hero's Pose (page 143) with padding under your hips, and root down and lengthen your spine. Draw your shoulders back to lift and open your chest, and place your hands on your knees with your thumbs and ring fingers touching, in what is called concentration mudra.

2 Place your right index and middle finger between your eyebrows, and place your right thumb on your right nostril and right ring finger on your left nostril (A). Close your eyes or keep them slightly open, and tune into the natural rhythm of your breath with your mouth closed, breathing in and out naturally though your nose.

3 Next, gently block off your right nostril with your thumb and inhale through your left nostril (B). Then block off your left nostril with your ring finger and release your thumb to breathe out through your right (C). Inhale right, switch, and exhale left. This counts as one full round. Again: Inhale left, switch, exhale right. Inhale right, switch, exhale left. Repeat for 3, 6, or 9 rounds, keeping the rhythm of the breath smooth and regulated through a count of 3 or 4.

4 As you focus on alternating nostrils, remember to keep doing your deep belly breathing at the same time!

5 When you're done, release your hands, keeping your head lifted and shoulders back.

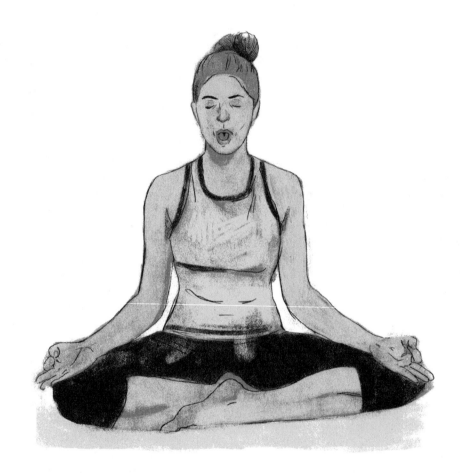

Cooling Breath

Sitali Pranayama

This breathing practice is both fun and funny looking! It soothes anxiety, anger, agitation, and stress. Once you get the hang of it, you can use this breath when you're overheated, overstimulated, overwhelmed, have insomnia, or need to chill out. It also helps curb thirst and hunger. There are two ways to practice this; if the first variation is not accessible, try the second.

1 Begin in Easy Pose (page 15) or Hero's Pose (page 143) with padding under your hips, and root down and lengthen your spine. Draw your shoulders back and open your chest. Place your hands palms up on your thighs with your thumbs touching your pinky fingers. This is a mudra that stimulates the water element in the body. Find a point of focus with your gaze in front of you, and tune in to the natural rhythm of your breath with your mouth closed, breathing in and out though your nose.

2 After a few breaths, make an O-shape with your lips to curl your tongue as you stick it out about ¾ inch, making it resemble a straw. Inhale through your tongue into your belly, draw your tongue back into your mouth, and exhale through your nose, contracting the lower ribs. Again, sip the breath in through your curled tongue and exhale through your nose. You'll feel a cooling sensation on your tongue as you inhale and a slight heating sensation on the exhale, tuning you in to the body's natural ventilation system.

3 If you can't curl your tongue, line up your top and bottom teeth and separate your lips. Breathe in through the gaps in your teeth and exhale through your nose. You will immediately feel the cooling air coming in, along with a little salivation, which is part of the hydrating and cooling process. Exhale through your nose.

4 Practice either variation in steps 2 and 3 for 3 to 5 minutes and pause to feel the cooling effects.

5

FIVE

Meditation Practice

"The thing about meditation is: You become more and more YOU."
—DAVID LYNCH

Meditation is at the heart of every yoga practice. Although incredibly beneficial on their own, asana and pranayama practices are meant to prepare the mind and body for meditation through concentration and focus. The benefits of meditation are believed to be vast, including reduced stress, deepened concentration, self-awareness, mindfulness, cardiovascular health, boosted immune system, and increased serotonin. The good thing about meditation is that you can do it anywhere and don't have to practice for hours on end to reap the benefits.

Meditation Techniques

Meditation is at its core the practice of training our minds by bringing our awareness to one singular point of focus. This sounds easy in theory, but can be difficult to practice. Our minds are constantly flowing from one thought to another. It's difficult to slow down and bring our focus to one single thing, or to be truly present in our lives and with the people we love. This is where meditation can help.

Meditation techniques include Insight Meditation, Transcendental Meditation, and Yogic Meditation. They all use different points of focus for the mind; you'll work out which type works best for you. The key to all meditation techniques is consistency. Meditating for 5 to 10 minutes every day is more beneficial than 30 to 60 minutes once a week.

The simplest meditation is to close your eyes and focus only on your breath. Draw your attention to every inhale and exhale. Every time you find your mind wandering, draw your focus back to the breath to get back in touch with yourself. Meditation is not about running away or escaping. It's about becoming more aware of our feelings, minds, and the world.

If you find that focusing on the breath is not enough to quiet your mind, you may come up with a mantra or intention that adds another layer to your meditation. This mantra can be a traditional Sanskrit mantra like the sound of *Om,* the sound of cosmic consciousness, it can also be *Om Shanti,* which means "peace." It can also be something you desire for yourself, for another, or for the world at large, like the word "love." By focusing on this mantra, not only are you creating a singular point of focus for your mind, but you're also sending the positive message out into the world.

If you're struggling with something in particular or need an extra point of focus, a guided imagery, visualization, or mudra can help. *Mudras* are sacred hand gestures, or yoga with your hands. These powerful gestures symbolize and awaken different spiritual qualities, such as compassion or courage, and are used for focus and intention in meditation practice. This type of meditation accesses the subconscious. Many athletes use this kind of visualization meditation when trying to achieve a certain feat. Guided imagery can be used for any type of challenge, such as anxiety, negative patterns or habits, illness or injury, or difficult relationships.

A Soothing Environment

While it's true that you can meditate anywhere at any time, this might not be possible as you begin the practice because of external distraction. Creating an assigned space to meditate will help you devote to and build your practice.

I like to set up a sacred environment for meditation wherever I am. When on the road, I bring my traveling altar to engage all my senses: a photo of my family, a candle, incense or fragrant oil, a bell, and *mala*, or prayer beads used for mantra repetition. As the mystic Joseph Campbell said, "Your sacred space is where you find yourself again and again."

You should never feel like you have to force yourself to meditate; it should be something you look forward to. Maybe you enjoy soft, soothing music to help drown out the city noises outside your window, or perhaps aromatherapy helps you physically relax. Incorporate whatever helps bring you inward.

Meditation, Mudra, and Mantra Practices

As you get started, first remind yourself that everyone's mind wanders during meditation. You'll need to be open and patient as you begin. The key is to dedicate yourself to your practice and try different techniques to find what works best for you. The following practices are a great way to start. Try them in order, gradually building up your daily meditation time. Choose a technique that really speaks to you and your intention to commit to daily practice. You can also adapt your practice slightly by choosing a different meditation daily to serve your needs at that time.

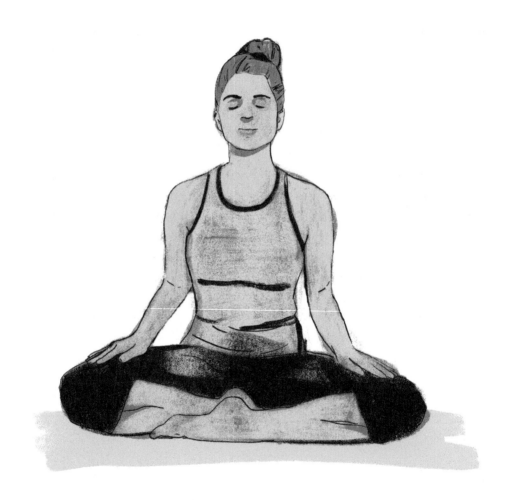

Buddha's Peaceful Abiding Meditation

This meditation is the most basic and simple one to practice daily to quiet and focus the mind. You want to focus on the breath and simply notice your thoughts, emotions, and sensations without judgment, and then let them go. A meditation cushion elevates you, making the position easier on the knees and hips. You can also use a folded blanket or even sit in a chair. To make sure your knees are in line with your hips and your spine is erect, either cross your legs or place your feet flat on the ground with your knees a few inches apart.

1 Place your hands on your thighs, sliding them back a little, and sit up tall with a strong back body and open, soft front with your shoulders back.

2 Soften your chin down a little to lengthen the back of your neck, and find a point of focus about 6 feet in front of you. Keep your eyes slightly open.

3 Keep your mouth slightly open with your tongue gently touching the roof of your mouth and breathe equally through the nose and mouth.

4 When you've established your seat, make an intention to create peace with your self, your life, and others by being with whatever arises.

5 Place your mind on your breath and keep it there as it moves in and out of your nose and mouth. When a thought arises, label it "thinking" as you exhale and return to noticing your breath as it goes in and out. This is a way of untangling your identity from your thinking and feelings and returning to the moment to be present with your breath and life.

6 Follow these instructions exactly. At first, this may be challenging, but after some time you may notice space and peace in the midst of the mind's chatter.

7 When your timer goes off, stretch your legs, and gradually return to your activities without rushing.

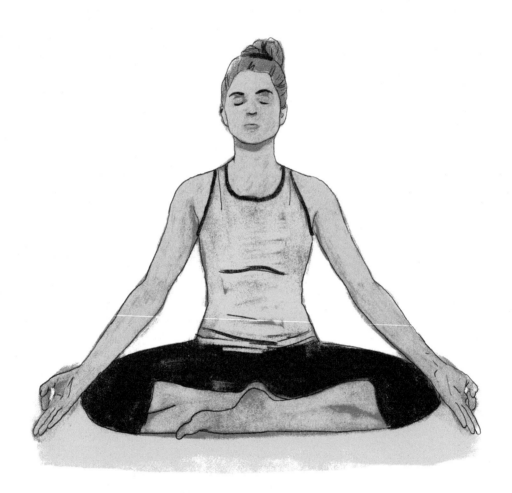

Yogi's Meditation

In this meditation, we focus on the sound of Om to develop greater concentration. In yogic texts, the sound of Om is said to be the universal sound that leads to union with the self. The intention of this practice is to cultivate inner union even amid all the changing forces of nature around us. Mantra repetition teaches us how we can transform our own thoughts from negative to positive, our moods from unhappy to happy, our lives from stressful to peaceful, and our habits from destructive to fulfilling.

1 Begin by following the steps for Buddha's Peaceful Abiding Meditation (page 229), creating a comfortable and steady seat, but place your hands on your knees and join your thumbs and index fingers together with the other 3 fingers extending toward the earth.

2 Close your eyes gently and turn your gaze in and up to the point between your eyebrows. This area is known as the third eye and is the Sixth Chakra, or spiritual energy center of concentration and intuition.

3 Inhale and then exhale *Om* silently and internally in your mind. If you notice your mind wandering, center it back on the mantra.

4 If you like, make the sound of *Om* 3 times aloud by inhaling deeply and exhaling to the sound—a long "o" ending with the "m" sound. The practice is meant to be done internally, so don't worry too much about the sound and remember you can do this meditation anywhere—even in a public place.

5 Practice this meditation before a longer basic meditation to focus your mind for 1 or 2 minutes, or 1 to 8 repetitions. You can also practice alone for 3 to 5 minutes.

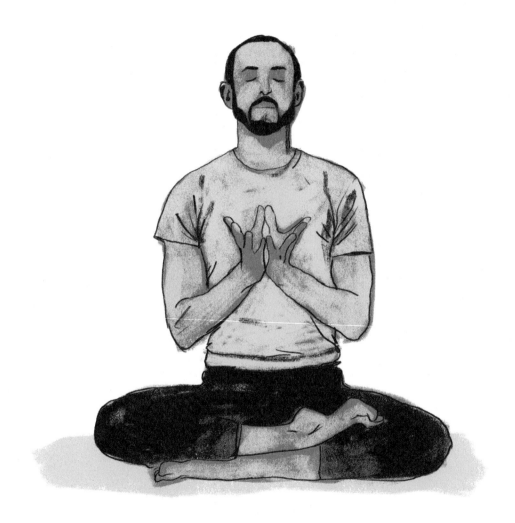

Cultivating Compassion Meditation

Compassion is at the heart of many spiritual traditions. It shifts our awareness away from ourselves, to wishing happiness for others. As the Dalai Lama says, "If you want others to be happy, practice compassion. If YOU want to be happy, practice compassion." This is great to practice any time you have feelings of grief, resentment, loneliness, anger, or sadness having to do with others.

1 Begin by following the basic instructions in Buddha's Peaceful Abiding Meditation (page 229). This time, place your hands in Lotus Mudra, and turn your gaze and focus toward your hands as though gazing at a beautiful flower. Place both hands in front of your heart with both your pinky finger side and thumb sides touching, with the base of your hands and your wrists forming a lotus flower. Spread your other fingers as wide as possible, keeping your pinkies, thumbs, and wrists together.

2 Take a few deep breaths as if smelling the most exquisite fragrance. The lotus grows within the mud but does not get one drop of mud on it. In the same way, we can be in the muddiness and muckiness of life but keep our hearts wide open.

3 Now begin the traditional Buddhist compassion practice of loving-kindness, or *maitri*. Start by sending out love and kindness with each exhale, first toward yourself, then toward people close to you like your family, then toward people who are more distant like your neighbors, then toward people you don't know who perhaps live in a different country, and lastly toward people who have caused you suffering. The last one can be quite challenging, but it is the highest form of liberation to keep our hearts open through forgiveness and by recognizing our shared humanity.

4 You can use the traditional mantra of "May _____ be free from suffering, may they experience health and happiness," or choose any kind words or prayers to send out to others.

5 After 3 to 5 minutes of this practice, release your hands to your thighs, and meditate on the joyful feelings released through this practice for another 5 minutes.

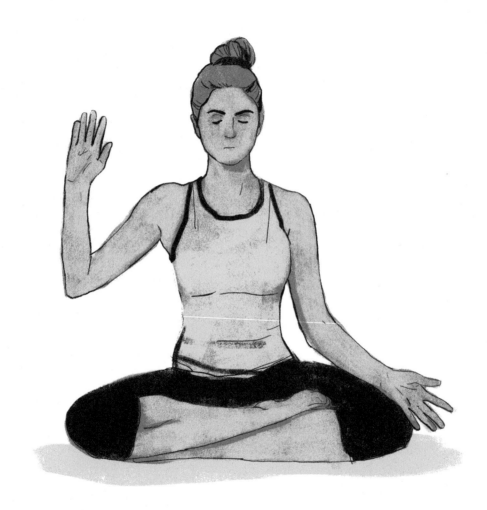

Cultivating Courage Meditation

In this meditation, you use the mudra of fearlessness—depicted in many Hindu and Buddhist paintings—to create a brave space in which to sit with difficulty. Cultivating the quality of courage is as important as peace or compassion in yoga. This quality allows you to face the many obstacles and fears of life nonviolently. Practice this meditation when you're struggling with any challenging situation and need to cultivate inner strength by confronting your fears.

1   Begin by creating a stable seat. Sit up tall with a strong back, cultivating the courage to keep your heart open and vulnerable. Place your left hand on your thigh and lift your right hand to the outside of your right shoulder, bending your elbow by your side.

2   Place your mind on your breath. Inhale and let in everything that is causing you fear in your life. Breathe into the feeling. Hold it in your chest for a moment and then let it go. Instead of running away or avoiding situations that cause suffering, we welcome them and even make friends with them. The key is to sit with everything as a way of facing our fears and developing the courage to be fully present. As the Tibetan meditation master Chogyam Trungpa Rinpoche said, "Smile at fear." So you can try that too!

3   Stay with the mudra, your breath, and your posture for 3 to 5 minutes with the intention to cultivate courage. Then release the mudra and come back to the basic meditation, resting in the bravery that was awakened through your practice. There is so much fear plaguing our world. This meditation is a powerful medicine at any time.

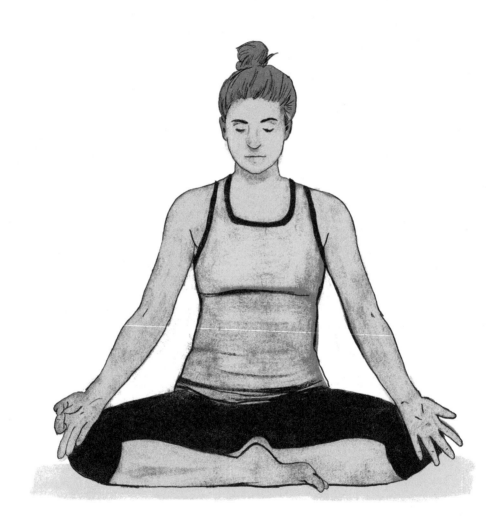

Earth Witness Meditation

This mudra simulates the Buddha's gesture on forgoing his final liberation to stay on Earth and serve others. In the same way, this meditation grounds and roots us to our worldly life. Use this meditation when you're having difficulty being present or lacking faith that everything is exactly as it should be. This is a great basic mindfulness meditation and mudra to practice daily for 10 to 30 minutes, especially in the morning. With the right hand rooting into the earth, you can sit up and be more present in your meditation. With your left hand open, you can receive the simple blessings available in every moment.

1   Begin in the basic meditation posture. Allow your shoulders to melt down your back, opening your chest, and keep your gaze toward the earth about 6 feet in front of you in your commitment to stay present and awake to life.

2   Touch the ground with your right fingertips, rooting them into the earth, and sit up tall. Place the back of your left hand on your left knee with your hand open toward heaven. Root down into the earth with your right hand, feeling your connection to every being, and inhale through your fingers to receive strength and nourishment. Exhale through your open left hand and surrender to the moment. Inhale receiving, exhale giving.

3   The Vietnamese zen master and activist Thich Nhat Hanh teaches a beautiful breathing and mantra practice that can be used with this meditation: "Breathing in, I know I am breathing in. Breathing out, I know I am breathing out. Breathing in, I calm body and mind. Breathing out, I smile. Dwelling in the present moment, I know this is the only moment."

6

SIX

Balanced Routines

"I believe that we learn by practice. Whether it means to learn to dance by practicing dancing or to learn to live by practicing living, the principles are the same." —MARTHA GRAHAM

Yoga is meant to be fluid. The practice involves poses, meditation, and developing a deep connection with your body. It's less about following a certain order of poses or doing each one perfectly, and more about self-reflection and becoming more in tune with your body, your life, and the wider world. The most wonderful thing about yoga is that you can adapt it to your body and circumstances.

In this chapter, I outline a variety of routines for you to choose from. No matter the time of day, how much time you have, or how you're feeling, you can find a routine that works for you. An important part of practice is sequencing—thinking about the unique qualities of each pose and how to string them together so they flow naturally and work for your body. I use the sequences of these routines all the time in my own practice and my classes. Feel free to do partial routines or adapt them as you get more comfortable. Bringing creativity to your practice will make it even more satisfying and personal to you.

Making Yoga Part of Your Daily Life

Beginning and sticking to a daily home yoga practice is one of the most empowering acts of self-care. Our practice asks us to take personal responsibility for our own physical, mental, and spiritual health. So how do you actually motivate yourself to practice? Where will you find the time? As one of my teachers used to say, "Magic is in the repetition."

Masters suggest that we start with a little every day or regularly, rather than for a long time once a week. Be sure to pick a practice you enjoy so you'll keep returning to it day after day. The most important thing is to adapt the practice to your life instead of adapting your life to your practice.

CARVE OUT A TIME

Figure out how much time you have and the best time to practice, and schedule that into your calendar. A few tips for success:

» Find a time of day that works best for you and try to stick to it without getting too attached.

» If you miss a day, just start again the next day or carve out 15 minutes later on. It's important to be flexible. Life is full of unpredictable twists and turns. Learning to adapt is one of yoga's highest teachings.

» You may choose to practice at a different time every day. The whole idea is to create *your* schedule and honor your life.

Your dosha (see page 25) can also help guide the best time of day to practice. Each dosha cycles twice in a day. You can align yourself with your dosha by practicing yoga during these times.

Pitta dosha: 10 a.m. – 2 p.m. and 10 p.m. – 2 a.m.

Vata dosha: 2 p.m. – 6 p.m. and 2 a.m. – 6 a.m.

Kapha dosha: 6 p.m. – 10 p.m. and 6 a.m. – 10 a.m.

CHOOSE YOUR PRACTICE

I've created three morning, three afternoon, and three evening balanced yogic routines of varying lengths. Each includes meditation and contemplation for the mind, movement for the body, and breathing for the spirit. This allows for an integrated, well-rounded practice.

VINYASAS

The routines in this chapter blend together Vinyasa Yoga and Hatha Yoga. Vinyasa is a flowing style that links the rhythm of the breath with the physical poses, which are strung together into a sequence. During these practices, you'll come across lists of poses together. Practice these "chains" of poses in order, first on the right side and then on the left, unless specified otherwise.

For Hatha Yoga, poses are held for longer periods of time. You'll see the time length for each pose noted in the steps.

The term "vinyasa" refers to a part of the Sun Salutation series (page 199) that includes a series of counter poses. A vinyasa is often practiced during a routine to reset the body before switching sides. You can leave this out of any routine if it feels too strenuous.

The following is the Basic Vinyasa often practiced with one breath per movement:

Downward-Facing Dog

Plank

Knees, Chest, Chin or Yogi's Push-Up

Baby Cobra or Upward-Facing Dog

Downward-Facing Dog

Practice the Basic Vinyasa a few times and memorize it, since it is central to many of the following routines.

If you have never practiced yoga before, be sure to start with the 15-to-30-minute routines until the movements become familiar. Then you will be ready to move on to the 30-to-45-minute routines that include different vinyasas. With some consistency, in a few months, you will be ready for the 60-to-75-minute routines. Feel free to adapt the practices to your body and stay with poses that you want to master.

In general, morning practices are more energizing, mid-day practices more balancing, and evening practices more calming. I've labeled each routine as *calming, balancing,* or *energizing,* and each one has unique healing qualities. Think of these routines as preparing healthy recipes: You put some effort into preparing a meal and then enjoy the delicious and wholesome result. In the same way, you'll need to dedicate time for your practice, and then you get to enjoy the blissful outcome throughout your day.

Before you choose your practice, check in with yourself about what you need. If you need a more calming practice in the morning because you have a stressful day ahead, feel free to choose a calming evening practice instead to start your day. After a week or so, you'll be able to choose poses you love and incorporate them into one of these practices, or even design your own practice.

BEGINNER'S SAMPLE PRACTICE

TIME: 15 to 30 Minutes

QUALITY: calming, grounding, balancing

Try the following starter routine to get you into the flow and to quiet your mind. You can even put on some relaxing music to inspire you. You should also practice the Warrior's Breath (page 215) throughout this routine and all the following ones for its powerful effects on the mind and body.

1 Deep Relaxation (page 183) with Simple Supine Belly Breath (page 213), 10 breaths

2 Supine Twist (page 157), 5 breaths on each side

3 Supine One-Leg Stretch (page 161), 5 breaths on each side

4 Child's Pose (page 35), 5 breaths

5 Cat-Cow (page 187), 5 rounds

6 Tibetan Sun Salutation (page 191), 5 rounds

Basic Vinyasa

7 Downward-Facing Dog (page 37), 3 breaths

8 Plank (page 39), 2 breaths

9 Knees, Chest, Chin (page 41), 1 breath

10 Baby Cobra (page 45), 2 breaths

11 Downward-Facing Dog, 3 breaths

12 Repeat Basic Vinyasa

13 Standing Forward Bend (page 51), hold on to either elbow and rock side-to-side, 3 breaths

14 Mountain (page 49), 5 breaths

15 Standing Forward Bend

16 Downward-Facing Dog

17 Child's Pose, 3 breaths

18 One-Leg Side Stretch Pose (page 169), 5 breaths each side

19 Goddess Pose (page 181), 8 breaths

20 Deep Relaxation, 3 to 5 minutes

21 Buddha's Peaceful Abiding Meditation (page 229), 3 to 5 minutes

MORNING
ROUTINES
ENERGIZING

In Ayurvedic and yogic wisdom, the morning hours of 6 a.m. to 10 a.m. are ruled by the Kapha dosha, or the energy of heaviness. No wonder we tend to feel sleepy and need that cup of coffee to get going! An energizing, invigorating, and faster paced practice is recommended in the morning, along with waking up as early as possible— even before 6! The morning routines that follow often contain a vinyasa between sides. They are all energizing and clear your mental fog.

GET UP AND GO

TIME: 15 to 30 minutes
QUALITY: Energizing

This will wake up your mind and body and get you moving right out the door. Flow from one pose to the next with the rhythm of your breath like a moving meditation.

1   Tibetan Sun Salutation (page 191) with Warrior's Breath, 5 to 8 rounds

Basic Vinyasa

2   Downward-Facing Dog (page 37), 3 breaths

3   Plank (page 39), 3 breaths

4   Knees, Chest, Chin (page 41), 1 breath

5   Baby Cobra (page 45), 2 breaths

6   Downward-Facing Dog

7   Crescent Moon (page 57), right leg, 3 breaths

8   Stoke the Fire (page 195)

9   Repeat Basic Vinyasa

10 Crescent Moon, left leg, 3 breaths

11 Repeat Basic Vinyasa

12 Standing Forward Bend (page 51), 3 breaths

13 Mountain (page 49), 3 breaths

14 Triangle (page 77), right side then left side, 3 breaths each side

15 Warrior II (page 67), right side then left side, 3 breaths each side

16 Powerful Pose (page 61), 3 breaths

17 Boat (page 113), 3 breaths

18 Half Wheel (page 149), 3 breaths

19 Supine Twist (page 157), right side, then left side, 3 breaths each side

20 Supine Pigeon (page 205)

21 Deep Relaxation (page 183), 3 minutes

22 Buddha's Peaceful Abiding Meditation (page 229), 3 minutes

RISE AND SHINE

TIME: 30 to 45 minutes
QUALITY: Energizing

This invigorating practice is perfect when you have a little more time to include breathing practices and meditation for your mind, and need an energizing but grounding physical practice. In this routine, standing poses link together into a vinyasa practice, flowing from one to the next.

1 Cleansing Breath (page 217)
2 Stoke the Fire (page 195)
3 Mountain (page 49)
4 Tree (page 99)
5 Powerful Pose (page 61)
6 Standing Forward Bend (page 51)

Basic Vinyasa

7 Plank (page 39)
8 Yogi's Push-Up (page 43)
9 Upward-Facing Dog (page 47)

Warrior Vinyasa (right side)

10 Warrior I (page 65)
11 Warrior II (page 67)
12 Peaceful Warrior (page 69)
13 Triangle (page 77)
14 Extended Side Angle (page 79)

15 Repeat Basic Vinyasa
16 Repeat Warrior Vinyasa, left side
17 Plank
18 Side Plank (page 115)
19 Downward-Facing Dog (page 37)
20 High Lunge (page 55), right side
21 Revolved Extended Angle (page 93), right side then left side
22 Forearm Plank (page 119)
23 Dolphin (page 129)
24 Headstand Prep (page 133)
25 Locust (page 145)
26 Bow (page 147)
27 Half Wheel (page 149)
28 Supine One-Leg Stretch (page 161)
29 Supine Twist (page 157)
30 One-Leg Side Stretch (page 169)
31 Deep Relaxation (page 183)
32 Yogi's Meditation (page 231)

CARPE DIEM (SEIZE THE DAY!)

TIME: 60 to 75 minutes
QUALITY: Energizing

Take about an hour to indulge in a deep, heating, purifying, and energizing practice to transform your day with twists and inversions. Great in the winter or when you need extra energy, or any time to feel like you could change the world!

1   Cultivating Courage Meditation (page 235)

2   Bellows Breath (page 219)

3   Cleansing Circles and Twists (page 189)

4   Stoke the Fire (page 195)

5   Mountain (page 49)

6   Full Sun Salutation (page 199)

7   Powerful Pose (page 61)

8   Standing Forward Bend (page 51)

Basic Vinyasa

9   Plank (page 39)

10 Yogi's Push-Up (page 43)

11 Baby Cobra (page 45)

12 Downward-Facing Dog (page 37)

Eagle Vinyasa (right side)

13 Warrior I (page 65)

14 Warrior II (page 67)

15 Standing One-Leg Balance (page 101)

16 Eagle Pose (page 105)

17 Repeat Eagle Vinyasa, left side

Rotated Vinyasa (right side)

18 High Lunge (page 55)

19 Revolved Extended Angle (page 93)

20 Revolved Half Moon (page 95)

21 Standing Forward Bend

22 Seated Spinal Twist (page 165)

23 Repeat Rotated Vinyasa, left side

24 Boat (page 113)

25 Crow (page 121)

26 L-Shaped Handstand (page 125) or Handstand (page 127)

27 Locust (page 145)

28 Bow (page 147)

29 Half Wheel (page 149)

AFTERNOON
ROUTINES
BALANCING

Midday is the best time to find balance, since the sun is at its highest point. This is the time of the Pitta dosha when we are naturally the most energized, but can also be depleted and overworked, worked up, and in need of a break to recharge. This is the time we should have our largest meal since the digestive fire is at its strongest, so your practice should be nourishing and replenishing. Practice sun salutations slower, and maybe leave out some of the vinyasas or practice them at a gentler level.

YOGI'S LUNCH BREAK

TIME: 15 to 30 minutes

QUALITY: Balancing

This hip-opening practice is nourishing and fulfilling before or after lunch, or any time.

1. Cooling Breath (page 223)
2. Cleansing Circles and Twists (page 189)
3. Cat-Cow (page 187)
4. Downward-Facing Dog (page 37)
5. Lizard Lunge (page 59), right side

Basic Vinyasa

6. Downward-Facing Dog
7. Plank (page 39)
8. Knees, Chest, Chin (page 41)
9. Baby Cobra (page 45), 2 breaths
10. Downward-Facing Dog

11. Lizard Lunge, left side
12. Repeat Basic Vinyasa
13. Mountain (page 49)
14. Tree (page 99)

Flowing Vinyasa (right side)

15. Warrior II (page 67)
16. Peaceful Warrior (page 69)
17. Triangle (page 77)
18. Extended Side Angle (page 79)
19. Half Moon (page 81)
20. Warrior II

21. Repeat Flowing Vinyasa, left side
22. Wide-Legged Forward Bend (page 83)
23. Warrior Goddess (page 73)
24. Garland (page 85)
25. Seated Pigeon (page 207)
26. Resting Pigeon (page 207)
27. Straddle Forward Bend (page 173)
28. Goddess (page 181)
29. Deep Relaxation (page 183)
30. Yogi's Meditation (page 231)

AFTERNOON PICK-ME-UP

TIME: 30 to 45 minutes

QUALITY: Balancing

This practice is a more uplifting afternoon one to refuel and get you through the rest of your day.

1 Cleansing Breath (page 217)

2 Tibetan Sun Salutation (page 191)

3 Stoke the Fire (page 195)

4 Mountain (page 49)

5 Powerful Pose (page 61)

6 Standing Forward Bend (page 51)

7 Crescent Moon (page 57), right side

Basic Vinyasa

8 Downward-Facing Dog (page 37)

9 Plank (page 39)

10 Knees, Chest, Chin (page 41)

11 Baby Cobra (page 45), 2 breaths

12 Downward-Facing Dog

13 Crescent Moon, left side

14 Downward-Facing Dog

15 Warrior I (page 65)

16 Humble Warrior (page 71)

17 Repeat Basic Vinyasa

18 Warrior I – Humble Warrior, left side

Cleansing Vinyasa (right side)

19 Pyramid Pose (page 89)

20 Revolved Triangle (page 91)

21 Standing Split (page 109)

22 Seated Spinal Twist (page 165)

23 Repeat Cleansing Vinyasa, left side

24 Dancer's Pose (page 107)

25 Boat (page 113)

26 Dolphin (page 129)

27 Forearm Stand (page 131)

28 Hero's Pose (page 143)

29 Locust (page 145)

30 Bow (page 147)

31 Half Wheel (page 149)

32 Supine Twist (page 157)

33 Supine One-Leg Stretch (page 161)

34 Full Forward Bend (page 175)

35 Cultivating Compassion Meditation (page 233)

36 Legs Up the Wall (page 179)

37 Deep Relaxation (page 183)

LOVE IN THE AFTERNOON

TIME: 60 to 75 minutes

QUALITY: Balancing

Like the perfect date, this routine includes time to ease in and take it slow. It includes meditation, breathing, physical, and relaxation practices to nourish and balance your body, mind, and spirit.

LOVE IN THE AFTERNOON (CONTINUED)

EVENING ROUTINES
GROUNDING AND CALMING

Evening classes at yoga studios are the busiest, filled with people wanting to shake off the day and decompress to prepare for a restful evening. These practices include more soothing move-ment for the nervous system, standing poses that are held longer, and forward bends to ground the restless mind. Mean-while, inversions reverse the flow of energy, and restorative poses, calming breathing prac-tices, and a long final relaxation all allow you to let go of the day.

BLISSFUL BEDTIME ROUTINE

TIME: 15 to 20 minutes

QUALITY: Grounding and calming

Enjoy this blissful bedtime routine. Like a soothing soak, it will dissolve tension from your body and mind for a restful sleep.

1 Simple Supine Belly Breath (page 213)

2 Supine Twist (page 157)

3 Supine One-Leg Stretch (page 161)

4 Child's Pose (page 35)

5 Cat-Cow (page 187)

6 Knees, Chest, Chin (page 41)

7 Baby Cobra (page 45)

8 Downward-Facing Dog (page 37)

9 Lizard Lunge (page 59), right side then left side

10 Standing Forward Bend (page 51)

11 Mountain (page 49)

12 Triangle (page 77)

13 Wide-Legged Forward Bend (page 83)

14 Garland (page 85)

15 Downward-Facing Dog

16 Locust (page 145)

17 Seated Pigeon (page 207)

18 Sage Twist (page 167)

19 One-Leg Side Stretch (page 169)

20 Straddle Forward Bend

21 Goddess (page 181)

22 Legs Up the Wall (page 179)

23 Buddha's Peaceful Abiding Meditation (page 229)

24 Deep Relaxation (page 183)

EVENING CHILL-OUT PRACTICE

TIME: 30 to 45 minutes

QUALITY: Grounding and calming

Nighttime rituals are essential to transition between a busy day and quiet night. No one knows this better than parents! In the same way we get the little ones to bed, we need time to unwind since it's hard for our nervous system to switch on its own. Grounding movement is essential to calm the mind and wring out tension from the organs and muscles. Restorative inversions wash away worries and breathing practices reconnect you to your spirit.

HAPPY HOUR

TIME: 60 Minutes
QUALITY: Calming and Grounding

After a challenging day, a full-hour practice is an ideal way to smooth the transition to your personal or family time and be able to be fully present. This is the perfect happy hour, and includes cleansing twists, flowing sun salutations, grounding standing poses, fun inversions, heart-opening backbends, the coolest cooldown, and mindfulness meditation.

7

SEVEN

Living Yoga Off the Mat

By now, I hope you've come to understand the incredible tradition of yoga and its life-transforming powers. Yoga is a lifelong spiritual practice that evolves over time, adapting to every phase of your life. My wish is for you to experience the many blessings of yoga for years to come.

Because yoga is a way of living, the practice goes well beyond the mat. You'll find that incorporating asanas, meditation, and breathing practices into your everyday life will start to affect your entire way of being. With conscious movement, breathing, and thinking comes conscious living, from the inside out.

Yoga Diet

Many yoga practitioners end up changing their diet once their practice becomes a significant part of their lives. This can be a subconscious change as you begin to listen to your body, like eating when you're hungry and stopping when you're full. Or you can consciously initiate a change. You may make some changes given a renewed desire to be healthier, or find inspiration in the Eight Limbs of Yoga (see page 16) or the Ayurvedic practices (see page 25). What you eat has a huge impact on your mind, body, and emotions. Some foods are energizing, increasing vitality and strength, while others sap our energy. The basic principle of yoga on and off the mat is to enter a state of harmony. In this way, eating is yoga.

A variety of diets are popular among yoga practitioners. You don't have to blindly follow any one diet to practice yoga. In thinking about your diet, remember that yoga teaches us how to eat for our own bodies, schedules, and personalities. You may choose to explore other diets or variations on these diets. The one general rule to follow is to learn to eat mindfully. This means taking the time to cook your own food. Enjoy each smell and savor each flavor. Slow down to listen to the cues of your body, discovering your intuition and tuning into your nutritional needs.

Here are some of the prevalent diets in the yoga world:

Vegetarian Eating no animals has been the traditional yogic diet though the centuries. This is based on the principle of ahimsa, which means, "do no harm." Some vegetarians eat dairy and eggs and occasionally fish, but their main diet is plant based.

Vegan The vegan lifestyle takes the practice of vegetarianism one step further, renouncing all animal products in food, clothing, and cosmetics as a way of life. Sticking primarily to fruits, veggies, grains, nuts, seeds, and legumes, the vegan diet may seem strict but is becoming a popular way of living and eating. The vegan diet benefits the body and the whole planet. Since yoga means "union," this can be an empowering way to see how your personal choices have the power to affect the world.

Ayurveda Ayurvedic eating focuses on adapting what we eat to our specific dosha or constitution (page 25), as well as seasonal changes. It is a varied diet focused on eating to all six tastes: sweet, salty, sour, pungent, bitter, and astringent. These tastes contain the elements used to balance your dosha. Eating seasonally is another simple Ayurvedic practice that encourages us to live in harmony with nature.

Raw With a raw food diet, no food is cooked at over 118°F. The theory behind eating raw food is that when food is cooked, essential enzymes are destroyed and we miss out on their benefits. Raw foodists eat uncooked, unprocessed, and mostly organic foods.

In the Classroom

While cultivating a daily home practice is essential, you might also want to incorporate classes into your routine. This way you can learn firsthand from a trained teacher and also experience the sense of community that comes from practicing with others. *Sangha*, or *Satsang*, "practicing together in community," is another important aspect of yoga.

It's normal to feel a little timid when attending a yoga class for the first time. But going to class is an exciting adventure. It's a great opportunity to widen your practice and connect with others.

If you do feel fearful or nervous, remind yourself that the goal of yoga is to honor your body. There is no competition in yoga, and no need to compare yourself to those around you. Your practice is your practice. Yoga is about being an eternal beginner. There are no advanced postures, only opportunities to be a beginner again. Good teachers honor this philosophy wholeheartedly and will support you right where you are.

You can find a class at the gym, the YMCA, a boutique studio, or a chain of studios. Explore your options. Try out different classes and teachers. Try out different styles. Find what works best for you. Just because you show up at a class once doesn't mean that you must go there forever. Know that there are many styles, classes, and teachers out there, and that as you evolve as a human and a yoga practitioner, your needs and preferences will change. Don't be shy about mixing it up. Following are some of the yoga styles you might want to explore.

Hatha Most yoga classes are a form of Hatha Yoga, which incorporates asana and pranayama to still the fluctuations of the mind. "Ha" means sun and "tha" means moon, referring to a union of the opposites within, such as: male/female, strength/flexibility, and effort/surrender. Generally slower moving and gentle, these classes are perfect for beginners and great for when you need to slow down and unwind.

Vinyasa or Flow This flowing, dynamic style of yoga coordinates movement with the rhythm of the breath as a moving meditation. Most Vinyasa classes incorporate music, meditation and other modalities as a creative contemporary style (I teach this style). These classes tend to have a faster and more dance-like pace than Hatha Yoga classes. They build heat, strength, and flexibility. Make sure to take a basic Vinyasa class before jumping in.

Ashtanga Developed by yoga master Pattabhi Jois, Ashtanga is practiced on a fixed schedule—6 days a week with 1 day of rest, also resting on full and new moon days. It includes a set series of Vinyasa Yoga. This is mainly done as a self-practice with a teacher who will assist you into the poses. This is a challenging and very disciplined traditional style of yoga that builds heat. The original type of "power" yoga, it's a physical and mental workout.

Kundalini Kundalini focuses on breath, movement, music, mantra, dance, and meditation. It's considered one of the most spiritual practices, and focuses on stirring up and moving the energy that exists at the base of the spine. With less physical movement and more powerful breath, mantra, and mudra work, this practice is great for when you need to shake up your normal routine. It calls on developing the will and challenges the mind with repetitions and meditations of up to 30 minutes. Practice Kundalini when you're feeling stuck!

Iyengar Developed by yoga master B. K. S. Iyengar, this system of yoga focuses on alignment and breath control. A type of Hatha Yoga, it's characterized by its great attention to detail and use of props. Unlike Vinyasa Yoga, poses are held for a long time, developing strength as well as flexibility. Iyengar is great for getting to know your body and for healing injuries.

Yin A more quiet, deep, and relaxing form of yoga, yin holds poses with the assistance of props for 3 to 5 minutes at a time. These poses are meant to open up the body and release any tension.

Restorative Sometimes dubbed "the class where you figure out how many different ways you can lie down in an hour," restorative yoga is a great way to end your day or week, or to practice when you're nursing an injury or are feeling run down. It also uses props to help your body reach a more relaxed state. This style is deeply therapeutic and healing.

All of these yoga styles vary in their instruction style and the sequence of poses. Yet they all work toward the goal of uniting the body and the mind and connecting you to your true self. No matter what type of practice you choose, you'll feel the benefits.

Taking Your Practice into the World

While we've focused on the ways yoga can help you develop positive habits for a calm mind, healthy body, and joyful spirit, one of the bigger benefits of yoga is how it can affect the world at large. There's that saying, "You can't really find love until you learn to love yourself." The same is true with yoga. By understanding your own body, mind, and emotions along with your needs, desires, shortcomings, accomplishments, strengths, and weaknesses, you'll start understanding those around you. Being able to connect with others and the world at a deeper level is one of the greatest gifts of yoga.

In many yoga practices, the teacher will invoke the students to engage in a round of chanting *Om*. *Om* is believed to be the sound of the universe, the unifier of all things. No matter what we look like, what we do, how much money we make, or our struggles, *Om* is the frequency with which we all vibrate.

When we understand that we're no different from anyone around us, we become a part of something bigger than ourselves.

Seva is a yogic term that means "selfless service," and is integral to every traditional path of yoga. This concept is about serving and giving to others not because we have more, but because we are all one. Although most people think yoga is a pacifist path, it's actually a path of peaceful action. As we fight for our own right to health, happiness, and harmony, we show up to fight for the equal rights of all.

Here are five simple ways to practice yoga off the mat and experience your connection to all:

1 Practice ahimsa, or nonviolence, with every thought, word, deed, and action. This is a way to become conscious of how we may inadvertently participate in destructive dynamics. By becoming aware of negative thinking and speech toward others (including gossip), the products we use, and what we consume, we can contribute to lessening the suffering of others. You can do this in small ways every day.

2 Be present while you're out in the world (meaning, spend less time on your phone!). This will help you connect to others. Make a conscious choice to make eye contact and smile, or even say "Hello." Just looking at the sky, the trees, the earth beneath your feet becomes a walking meditation. As Thich Nhat Hanh says, "Walk as if with each step, your feet are kissing the earth."

3 Choose a specific cause as part of Karma Yoga, the yoga of self-transcendent action. There are so many causes to contribute time or money to. All that matters is that you choose one and give selflessly from the heart. In the end, you'll receive so much from giving!

4 Living a simple life that has the least negative impact on our planet is living yoga. Learn to discern between want and need. Do you really *need* the newest iPhone or jeans? Buying recycled clothes and products is a great way to reduce waste. Donate everything you don't need to charities. Conserve water, turn off lights, and unplug appliances. Buy local food and support small businesses. These are all practices of being one with others for the benefit of all.

5 Step outside your small social circle and neighborhood. Meet people from different cultures, classes, and religions. Engage in the world in a bigger way, and broaden your perspective to deepen your life experience.

The beautiful Indian greeting, "Namaste," which I say at the end of every practice, means "The divine light in me bows to the divine light in you." It's the recognition that we all share the experience of being human as well as divine. When we can connect to that, we are practicing yoga, and that is the greatest gift of all.

APPENDIX
YOGA LIBRARY

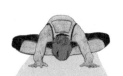

Alternate Nostril Breath
Nadi Shodhana Pranayama
(page 221)

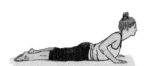

Baby Cobra Pose
Bhujangasana (page 45)

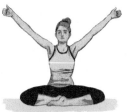

**Bellows Breath
(Breath of Fire)**
Bhastrika Pranayama (page 219)

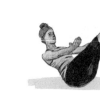

Boat Pose
Navasana (page 113)

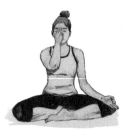

Bound Angle Pose
Baddha Konasana
(page 171)

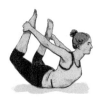

Bow Pose
Dhanurasana
(page 147)

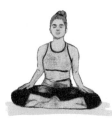

**Buddha's Peaceful
Abiding Meditation**
(page 229)

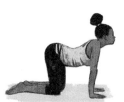

Cat-Cow (Cow)
Marjaryasana-Bitilasana
(page 187)

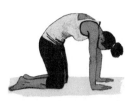

Cat-Cow (Cat)
Marjaryasana-Bitilasana
(page 187)

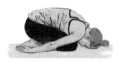

Child's Pose
Balasana (page 35)

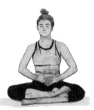

Cleansing Breath
Kapalbhati Pranayama
(page 217)

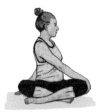

Cleansing Circles
and Twists
(page 189)

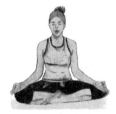

Cooling Breath
Sitali Pranayama (page 223)

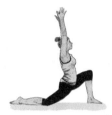

Crescent Moon Pose
Anjaneyasana (page 57)

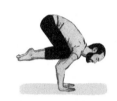

Crow Pose
Bakasana (page 121)

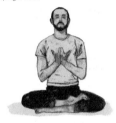

Cultivating Compassion
Meditation
(page 233)

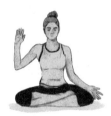

Cultivating Courage
Meditation
(page 235)

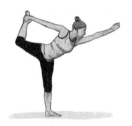

Dancer's Pose
Natarajasana (page 107)

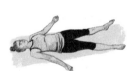

Deep Relaxation Pose
Savasana (page 183)

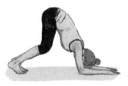

Dolphin Pose
Ardha Pincha Mayurasana
(page 129)

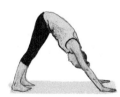

Downward-Facing
Dog Pose
Adho Mukha Svanasana (page 37)

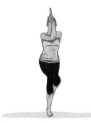

Eagle Pose
Garudasana (page 105)

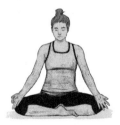

Earth Witness Meditation
(page 237)

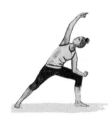

Extended Side
Angle Pose
Utthita Parsvakonasana (page 79)

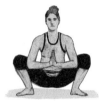

Forearm Plank Pose
Phalakasana (page 119)

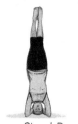

Forearm Stand Pose
Pincha Mayurasana (page 131)

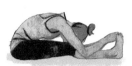

Full Forward Bend Pose
Paschimottanasana (page 175)

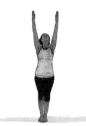

Full Sun Salutation
Surya Namasakara (page 199)

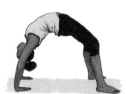

Full Wheel Pose
Urdhva Dhanurasana (page 151)

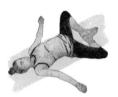

Garland Pose
Malasana (page 85)

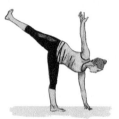

Goddess Pose
*Utkata Konasana
(page 181)*

Half Moon Pose
Ardha Chandrasana (page 81)

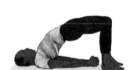

Half Wheel Pose
Setu Bandhasana (page 149)

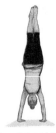

Handstand Pose
*Adho Mukha Vrksasana
(page 127)*

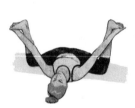

Happy Baby Pose
*Ananda Balasana
(page 159)*

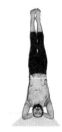

Headstand Pose
Sirsasana (page 135)

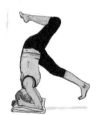

Headstand Prep Pose
*Ardha Sirsasana
(page 133)*

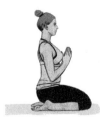

Hero's Pose
Virasana (page 143)

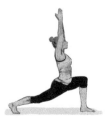

High Lunge Pose
*Utthita Ashwa Sanchalanasana
(page 55)*

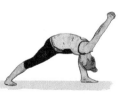

Humble Warrior Pose
*Virabhadrasana Bhakti
(page 71)*

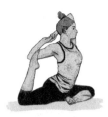

King Pigeon Pose
*Eka Pada Rajakapotasana
(page 153)*

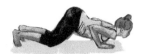

Knees, Chest, Chin Pose
*Ashtanga Namaskara
(page 41)*

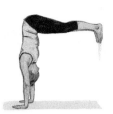

L-Shaped
Handstand Pose
*Adho Mukha Vrksasana
(page 125)*

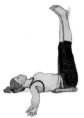

Legs Up the Wall Pose
Viparita Karani (page 179)

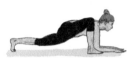

Lizard Lunge Pose
Utthan Pristhasana (page 59)

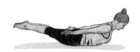

Locust Pose
Shalabhasana (page 145)

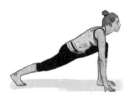

Low Lunge Pose
Anjaneyasana (page 53)

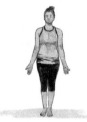

Mountain Pose
Tadasana (page 49)

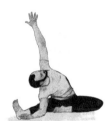

One-Leg Side
Stretch Pose
*Parivrtta Janu Sirsasana
(page 169)*

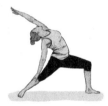

Peaceful Warrior Pose
*Virabhadrasana Shanti
(page 69)*

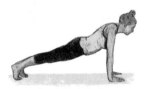

Plank Pose
*Utthita Chaturanga Dandasana
(page 39)*

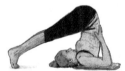

Plow Pose
Halasana (page 137)

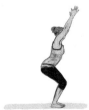

Powerful Pose
Utkatasana (page 61)

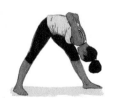

Pyramid Pose
Parsvottanasana (page 89)

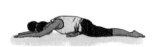

Resting Pigeon
*Eka Pada Kapotasana
(page 207)*

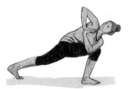

Revolved Extended
Angle Pose
*Parivrtta Parsvakonasana
(page 93)*

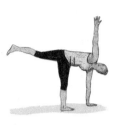

Revolved Half Moon Pose
Parivrtta Ardha Chandrasana
(page 95)

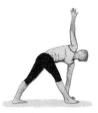

Revolved Half Moon with a block
Parivrtta Ardha Chandrasana
(page 95)

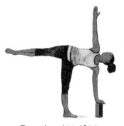

Revolved Triangle Pose
Parivrtta Trikonasana
(page 91)

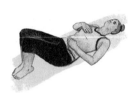

Sage Twist Pose
Bharadvajasana
(page 167)

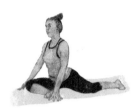

Seated Pigeon
Eka Pada Kapotasana (page 207)

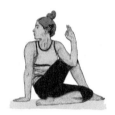

Seated Spinal Twist Pose
Ardha Matsyendrasana
(page 165)

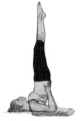

Shoulder Stand Pose
Salamba Sarvangasana
(page 139)

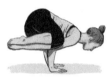

Side Crow Pose
Parsva Bakasana (page 123)

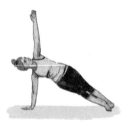

Side Plank Pose
Vasisthasana (page 115)

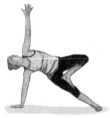

Side Plank with Tree Pose
(page 117)

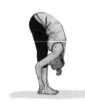

Simple Supine Belly Breath
(page 213)

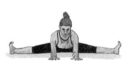

Standing Forward Bend Pose
Uttanasana (page 51)

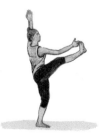

Standing One-Leg Balance Pose
Utthita Hasta Padangusthasana
(page 101)

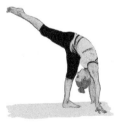

Standing Split Pose
Urdhva Prasarita Eka Padasana
(page 109)

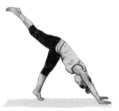

Stoke the Fire Pose
(page 195)

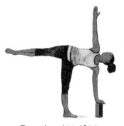

Straddle Forward Bend Pose
Upavistha Konasana (page 173)

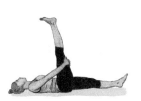

Supine One-Leg
Stretch Pose
Supta Padangusthasana
(page 161)

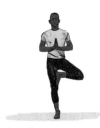

Supine Pigeon Pose
Supta Kapotasana
(page 205)

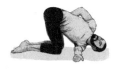

Supine Twist Pose
Supta Ardha Matsyendrasana
(page 157)

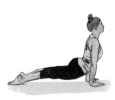

Thread the Needle Pose
Sucirandhrasana (page 193)

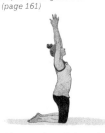

Tibetan Sun Salutation
Surya Namaskara (page 191)

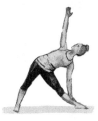

Tree Pose
Vrksasana (page 99)

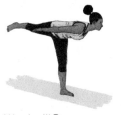

Triangle Pose
Trikonasana (page 77)

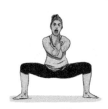

Upward Facing Dog Pose
Urdhva Mukha Svanasana
(page 47)

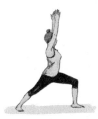

Warrior I Pose
Virabhadrasana I (page 65)

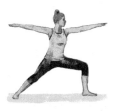

Warrior II Pose
Virabhadrasana II (page 67)

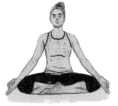

Warrior III Pose
Virabhadrasana III (page 103)

Warrior Goddess Pose
Shakti Asana (page 73)

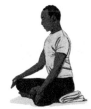

Warrior's Breath
Ujjayi Pranayama
(pages 17, 215)

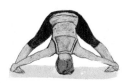

Wide-Legged
Forward Bend
Prasarita Padottanasana
(page 83)

Yogi's Meditation
(page 231)

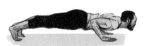

Yogi's Pushup Pose
Chaturanga Dandasana
(page 43)

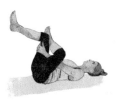

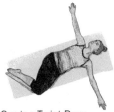

RESOURCES

These are some of my favorite yoga books, articles, videos, and resources to help and inspire you on your yoga journey.

BOOKS AND ARTICLES

Chodron, Pema. *How to Meditate: A Practical Guide to Making Friends With Your Mind.* Louisville, CO: Sounds True, 2013.

Desikachar, T. K. V. *The Heart of Yoga: Developing a Personal Practice.* Rochester, VT: Inner Traditions International, 1995.

Gannon, Sharon, and David Life. *Jivamukti Yoga: Practices for Liberating Body and Soul.* New York: Ballantine, 2002.

Farhi, Donna. *The Breathing Book: Good Health and Vitality Through Essential Breath Work.* New York: Holt, 1996.

Farhi, Donna. *Yoga Mind, Body, and Spirit: A Return to Wholeness.* New York: Holt, 2000.

Feuerstein, Georg, and Stephan Bodian. *Living Yoga: A Comprehensive Guide for Daily Life.* New York: Tarcher/Putnam, 1993.

Hirschi, Gertrude. *Mudras: Yoga in Your Hands.* San Francisco: RedWheel/Wieser, 2000.

Iyengar, B. K. S. *Light on Yoga.* New York: Schocken Books, 1979.

Iyengar, B. K. S. *Light on Pranayama.* New York: Crossroads Publishing, 2013.

Long, Ray. *The Key Muscles of Yoga: Your Guide for Functional Anatomy in Yoga.* Baldwinsville, NY: Bandha Yoga Publications, 2005.

McGreevey, Sue. "Eight Weeks to a Better Brain." *Harvard Gazette.* January 21, 2011. www.news.harvard.edu/gazette/story/2011/01/eight-weeks-to-a-better-brain/

The Meaning of "Yoga." www.yogajournal.com/article/beginners/the-roots-of-yoga/

Mehta, Silva, Mira Mehta, and Shyam Mehta. *Yoga the Iyengar Way: The New Definitive Illustrated Guide.* London: Dorling Kindersley, 1990.

Mipham, Sakyong. *Turning the Mind Into an Ally.* New York: Riverhead Books, 2003.

Schiffman, Erich. *Yoga: The Spirit and Practice of Moving into Stillness.* New York: Pocket Books, 1996.

Yee, Rodney. *Yoga: The Poetry of the Body.* New York: Thomas Dunne Books, 2002.

CLASSES AND COURSES

Laughing Lotus Yoga Centers: Laughinglotus.com

Integral Yoga Institutes: Integralyoga.org

VIDEOS

Yoga Anytime: Yogaanytime.com

Gaia's All Yoga videos: Gaia.com/yoga/practices

INDEX

ACKNOWLEDGMENTS

I'm am so very grateful to the following people for their support in making my lifelong dream of writing a yoga book come true.

First and foremost, thank you to Meg Ilasco and the entire Callisto Publishing team for this awesome opportunity and your incredible patience and persistence throughout the process.

Thank you to my husband, Raoul Ollman, for your steadfast support and belief in me, contributing your photographic skills for the book's images, and for being on overtime toddler duty.

Immense gratitude and love to my daughter, Indigo, for putting up with my long work days and lost weekends.

I couldn't have done this book without my sister, Ariana Tarkeshi, and my manager, Mario Batres, who ran Laughing Lotus Yoga Center while I took time off to write. Thank you, also, to all the teachers who jumped in to help.

Thanks to Mario and Robin Wilner for being my yogi models for the photographs. Marianne Velonis, thank you for your third eye on my writing. Thanks to Cory Martin for all of your writing support.

I extend deep gratitude to all my yoga and meditation teachers. There are way too many of you to name, but special thanks to Dana Flynn, Sarah Tomlinson, and Sharon Gannon for guiding me on my path these past 25 years and making this book possible. Thanks for introducing me to the ancient practices of yoga, which teach me every day how to show up and be a better person.

A very special thank-you to my mother, Alice Tarkeshi, for introducing me to the path of mindfulness 35 years ago. Thank you for continuing to teach me by the way you live each moment.

And finally, to all of YOU: Thank you for your interest in yoga. My students and readers are my greatest inspiration. Without you there would be no book.

ABOUT THE AUTHOR

JASMINE TARKESHI was named one of the 100 Most Influential Yoga Teachers in America in 2016. She has been teaching yoga for 20 years and has written articles for *Yoga Journal*, *Common Ground*, and *Body & Soul*, and has been quoted in and interviewed for numerous other publications including the *New York Times*, *Elle*, and the *San Francisco Chronicle*. She co-founded Laughing Lotus Yoga Centers in 1999 in New York City and San Francisco. She lives in San Francisco, California, with her husband, Raoul, and their daughter, Indigo, and close to her mother, Alice, and sister, Ariana.

CPSIA information can be obtained
at www.ICGtesting.com
Printed in the USA
BVOW05s1414060317
477413BV00001B/1/P